SKINCRAVE
TALES OF AN ADDICT

WRITTEN BY:

M.K. RAVE

ISBN: 978-1-960136-57-2

M.K.,

~~My Dearest Lover Boy~~

Here is a little booklet to jot down some ideas thoughts or feelings whenever you please. I was wanting you to lean towards using this as a goal, journal for your creative expression and me as a muse. I want to be your cheerleader for whatever dream you have for yourself I believe in you and I know you can make anything come true.

Introduction

Addict:

one exhibiting a compulsive, chronic, physiological, or psychological need for a habit-forming substance, behavior, or activity.

Well, I can tell you that my impulse to act on my wild thoughts formed many behaviors that led to many physiological needs. One of which was my favorite activity— SEX. Yes, I am a Love and Sex addict. Love story after love story fueled by substance abuse and unresolved trauma, the sex and love I would beg for would have me begging to end it all. Not all who identify as addicts make it out alive or bear the thought of telling the truth. I did. The labyrinth that is my road to recovery doesn't leave out the grimy details of how I survived to tell you that *Skincrave* is relevant, even if you don't con your way into getting what you want. This is my testimony of how I found my self-worth and spiritual body to save my life. The dirt that is my addiction tried to bury me alive, only to pile beneath me to help me climb out.

Imagine uncovering the life you grew up with, everything you were taught, how you were wired, and how you behaved, were the very things that led to your downfall. Becoming an addict wasn't what I had aspired to be, nor would I want to pass that on to the next generation. Still, I would learn the role my genetics and environment played as variables for this undoubtedly harsh reality. All the gestures I was programmed with would unravel at the seams when I found my voice outside of the ploy that is a "well-behaved woman." Saying yes to everything would finally lead me to my NO. This book is about uncovering what I didn't know about myself, under the covers. As a strong Latina woman, I am compelled to reveal my sex and love addiction, unapologetically, to show the process of how I was shaped into an addict and fought for my recovery with all the odds against me.

Content Warning

The names associated with my story have been changed to protect the privacy of those involved. Subjects addressed throughout the book can be triggering for some, and although the book is written with a certain hostility, I fully acknowledge the sensitivity of each event. Necessary caution is advised in efforts to protect the reader and their mental health around said subjects: drug use, blood, self-harm, suicide, death, eating disorders, sexual abuse, incest, miscarriage/abortion, and explicit sex.

#wellmannered

It's been said that you are either coming out of a storm, in the midst of a storm, or headed for one. What happens when you are the storm? A 5 '5, curvy, almond-eyed, plush-lipped storm. My parents would have done right by me, to name me Stormy. For now, I'll just go by M.K., and I am an addict. Have you ever known an addict? Or are you possibly the one who is addicted? I believe we are all creatures that harbor addictive tendencies; however, some of us don't escape unscathed by the drugs we choose to play with. My life is a composition made up of both active addiction and recovery, and no matter how carefully curated my words are, there is no getting past the nasty facts of each story. To be honest, I'm not trying to. I believe that if it weren't for me addressing the time I acted out of impulse to hurt myself or someone else, I wouldn't be here to tell my side of the story.

My drug of choice wasn't just snorting lines or drinking straight from the bottle when I should have just used a glass, since it's more socially acceptable; NO. My drug of choice was people. My first round of addictive behavior came from getting attention. Shit is harder to kick than sugar. Do you know what else is hard to stop? Sex. Someone once told me that I could go my whole life without using a drug ever again, but could I really go without ever having sex again? It dawned on me that I had labeled substance abuse as the only killer in people's homes and out on the streets. I would be sorely mistaken when my own love affairs would tragically end in death, right in the comfort of my own cushioned world. How could sex possibly kill anyone? But look at Romeo and Juliet, Othello, and King David in the Bible (2 Samuel

11:1-12:19). It was all relevant for the drama that would unfold in my life with a common denominator of sexual jealousy at the center, a tale as old as time.

To control such a primitive jolt in the mind is like asking a toddler not to choose candy over carrots. I tattooed the words Sexual Jealousy on the inside of my thighs because I understood the power I held as a female. The power I would abuse to get my way. Sex and love addiction is just as dangerous as any other addiction with how complex it is to identify with. I regret not speaking up about what I was experiencing. Allow me to uncover how I would use my looks and body for attention and create a world around sex that would leave scars more apparent than the tattoos on my face. No one told me how cliche I was acting by cashing in on my "beauty" everywhere I went, and if they did, it's not like I was listening. I was too busy riding the high of objectification. Craving a warm body would be my vice to mend my broken heart, only to land me in the lap of someone I would hate, over and over again. Or was it someone I loved? I couldn't tell the difference. There I was, lined up to do anything or anyone to get a high, whether I wanted it or not. That's the thing about addiction - once you start, it feels impossible to stop.

Riveting right? Before you roll your eyes, don't give me all the credit for being stereotypical. The skin crave I experienced for men and women alike isn't some groundbreaking discovery. It's not like I'm special or anything when in fact 18-24 million Americans have a sex addiction according to The National Council on Sexual Addiction Compulsivity. Dr. Stephanie Carnes, President of the International Institute for Trauma and Addiction, would remind me how I was one of the 80% of women who had become addicted to porn and most likely to act out on it. Who wants to admit that? ME. I'm bold enough to talk about it—no matter who I offend. It's the tragedy that comes after we use it that leaves a unique impression on our lives. It impacts us forever; enough to change some of us. Being nine years old and losing my virginity to a female family member isn't the story I thought I would ever have to tell. None of these obscene stories I'm about to share were stories I thought I could claim as my own, possibly considering them as made-up stories in my mind. Working through childhood trauma was the greatest decision I could've made for myself so I didn't have to walk around with my God complex any longer. Left to my own devices, things got ugly. There is a hope that I can help someone by saying what others won't. We are only as sick as our secrets, right?

The journey of short stories I'm about to take you on consists of raw, unadulterated truths about my relationships and how I used love and sex as my drug. I believe it is the grimy depth that can be brought to light to show people they don't have to stay in the dark. I no longer live in shame, and anyone who has used sex as a weapon shouldn't have to either. Giving myself a chance to put down all the weight I was carrying was how I was able to walk away and start living, not just surviving. I had been convinced to steer clear of saying anything that wasn't "ladylike" to keep being a well-mannered, proper woman. How's this for well-mannered? Pardon fucking me, but I'm talking now so politely shut the fuck up and let me speak. My voice had always been muffled out by the sounds of others speaking at me and not to me. Not anymore. That would all change and I would be the break in the cycle. I'm not against being kind or polite, or even stepping into my soft, feminine power when the time and place calls for it; but coerced into being the afterthought just because I am a woman isn't something I will let happen to me, again.

The truth looks different for everyone and no matter how you slice it, everyone seems to get a piece they don't appreciate. There are plenty of mixed feelings about the "truth" and whether or not it should be said, or how it should be delivered, but I am not in the business of sugarcoating. I have done my best to speak my piece without appeasing those around me, and protecting the feelings of those closest to me is long over. Some would say I'm oversharing and cringe at me for making waves, while others would still cringe but nod in approval for sharing the harsh truth. I vowed I would tell the truth for once, even if it wasn't to their face, so here it is...here's the truth.

Table of Contents

Chapter 1

#I'mGay#UreGay#let'sallbegay

It was 20__... you know, I just can't remember what year it was, so who gives a shit? Psychiatrists say trauma has a lasting side effect of amnesia. Evidence would claim it was a time in my life when everything ran together like the tattoos on my olive skin. And I am covered. I was okay with not knowing what was going on around me for the simple reason that I would have had to claim, at the very least, some responsibility for what had happened. Ew. Who wants that? What I do remember is I had already been married to a bisexual man named Christian, at 19 years old, and left him for multiple people, only to end up in the looney bin to recover from all the characters I was trying to be for all of my lovers. Quite the statement, right? "Victims" is what I'm told they were. I'm the victim if you ask me. If you also ask me where the best damn biscuits and gravy are served, I'd tell you the Northwest Pavilion Psychiatric Hospital. Why do mental institutions serve better food than grade school? Anyway, all I knew was that I was ready to leave after my weekend getaway for my suicide attempt. How did I get to that point? It started when I was a child, but we will get to that later.

I met Christian when I was 17 and he was my best friend! He was a wild, country boy from Texas and I couldn't resist the color of his eyes and how perfectly aligned his teeth were. I have a thing for teeth. Let's not forget that southern twang and the fact that he liked to suck dick! It was an attraction I felt was important to note because it would later determine how I profiled men. I noticed it wasn't the norm - being attracted to males who were attracted to males - and I never thought marrying a bisexual man was on my radar, but it was. Christian was perfect for me. He spiced up my life so much that I would now be able to check off the many boxes of dangerous living. My first, and last time, taking Xanax while handcuffed to a chair and being sexually aroused was with Christian. Jello-shots, raving, and rolling around shot-gun in his car while he played white-boy gangster was all in a day's work. I had graduated from homeschooling at 17 so I had all the time in the world to run away with this guy. My parents fucking hated him and it made me love him all the more. My loyalty to Christian came with a flagrant disregard for anyone or anything else in my life.

It was in Yellow, TX, which also happens to be where I was born and partially raised, that I started my rowdy lifestyle with Christian. I had to ping-pong back and forth between two states just to have time with each parent before I was old enough to be on my own. I made sure I had someone around to take care of my needs once I left home since all I had at the time was the 1995 Firebird my grandfather had given me for my 16th birthday and some birth control in my back pocket. Christian Mcall was the life of the party and had proven he would do absolutely anything for me, so he would do just fine as my husband. I tagged Christian as the man to take care of me because I thought that that's just what people do. Leave home, find their person, get married, and have them take care of you until you die. Fuck taking care of yourself, right?

Oh, how I wished I'd known differently. It's not like my dreams were to get into a good college that my parents stowed money away for, or backpack through Europe to gain a sense of culture outside my own. No. Why would I want my aspirations to be bolstered with knowledge and self-worth or the guidance and direction to pursue anything outside of my codependency? No, not crucial at all to teach me about finances or how the world works outside of my self-centered thinking, right?! I'll bash my parents more later but for now….My prerogative was to have fun and find someone to take care of me so I could have fun. And, boy did we have fun! Once we were at the happy, legal age of 18, we decided to have a courthouse wedding that my father would later find out about by reading the local newspaper. How the hell would I have known that nuptial ceremonies were printed in the local newspaper? I only opened a newspaper to read my horoscope and learn what my lucky numbers were for the day. As much as I downplayed the legality of what I had done, my dad would bring his true feelings to my attention by stating, "I want to shoot Christian in the kneecaps M.K." Seriously. Verbatim. There was no downplaying my dad's anger.

After tying the knot and staining the family name with such abrupt, foolish decisions, we knew it was time to buckle down and attempt to get their support by enrolling at a local college. What better way to win my family over than to behave like the overachiever I was in academics? I couldn't speak for Christian, but I wanted to start learning something outside of being drunk and high, and I was willing to do anything to get my family's approval of Christian despite all his scheming activities. We gave it the good old college try before Christian enlisted in the military. Before he left for basic training, we made sure to cause a stir and break our vows to one another. It was when Christian and I decided to bring outsiders into our relationship to keep the excitement going, that we soon learned how complicated we could make things between us. It seemed harder to find a male for our threesomes than to find a female so we kept the hunt narrowed in for the girls at our school. I felt like I was well versed with females, since I was a female, and it wasn't hard to befriend someone our age that was appealing to the naked eye with a soft-spoken attitude. Christian taught me that we wanted the hot chicks with low self-esteem because they were the ones who would do anything for attention. Whatever that meant. I was naive and wanted to please my now-husband, showing I would heed his every word, so I did what he said. I found us some candidates in hopes that they wouldn't spot we were up to no good. We were definitely no good and had no plan to stop.

I was looking for someone easy to get along with and who loved to party. Essentially, I was looking for someone like me. Aside from being loud, arrogant, and convincing; I needed to portray someone gentle and enticing in order to fluff the person we chose to invite to our sex party. My charismatic tone helped seal the deal every time. For instance, I had been in contact with a childhood friend of mine named Kaycee Lopez, who I remembered having a crush on my dad after she went on a ride along with him in his squad car. That's the sort of thing you can't forget; the possibility that one of your friends is banging your dad. Yuck! Before we were friends, I was her bully. Kaycee seemed to have forgiven me when I would bring her home to have a night she would never forget. It was luring people in that got me off more than the act of sex itself. I fell in love with the chase. I'm sure you've heard it said before that hunting as a predator can be better than catching the prey. I was a catch-and-release kind of chick, for the most part, but it was the deep abyss of attracting people that I got lost in. My options seemed limitless and my addiction began to form. After an evening of drinking and getting high, Kaycee landed on my bed making out with Christian. I watched them race each other to take off their clothes when I got the brilliant idea to run to the kitchen and grab a bomb-pop popsicle out of the freezer to take back to the bedroom as amo to go in for the kill. I loved using props in the bedroom.

Once I made it back to the loft where our mattress lay on the floor with no bedframe and Christmas lights accenting our walls to set the mood, I saw Kaycee on her back and Christian fingering her while lying next to her. I walked slowly towards the bed and dropped the popsicle on Kaycee's torso before it melted all over my hand. Why would I care if it melts? I was about to be covered with both Kaycee and red, white, and blue sugar. I took my time making her quiver knowing she felt both cold from the ice and the warmth of my tongue. Leaving lasting impressions was more important to me than first impressions. Kaycee once hated me; now she's in my bed. There wasn't any popsicle left for me to suck up, so I let Christian mount her. He definitely didn't practice any tantric discipline since it was a few pumps in before it was over. He claimed it was new and exciting so he couldn't hold it in. I didn't discredit that, but I would have enjoyed watching for longer, just as I'm sure Kaycee would have enjoyed him throbbing for longer. It was then and there that I knew I was a voyeur. Sure, I was disappointed I didn't get a turn with my own husband, but I can't blame the guy for not having the stamina for two slippery vixens. We politely sent Kaycee on her way and felt like our tag-teaming was impeccable. This is how love should be! Free to explore and not confined to a box. Chasing sexual fulfillment and pushing the limits was the only interest I had. How could this kind of love possibly end badly? Famous last words, right?

Here's what I knew so far: I loved watching my man have sex with other women and men, and I loved playing Cupid. It was so natural for me to push people's curiosity and organize an orgy. This was a dangerous skill, I know, but I couldn't help but lean into it. I also had a knack for getting too drunk and fighting with Christian. We were as toxic as it gets and this was one of many examples of how I thrived in chaos. If there wasn't the violence of throwing shit at each other or cops being called, was it even passionate love? If it wasn't the best sex of my life or spontaneous adventures with sex included, I didn't want it. Christain and I were always getting ourselves into trouble and it was hard to break away from it until he left for basic training for the army. I was forced to quit Christian cold turkey. Luckily for me, I had developed plenty of side relationships to keep me going while he was away. Some he knew about, some he didn't. Christian loved me in the most unhealthy way, but I knew that; I didn't care. I appreciated his unhealthy love until I couldn't see it, feel it, or have it when I wanted it. With him not around, all concepts of love fled like cockroaches in the light– exposed and running. I realized I was exposed without him and I had to run to find comfort. It was a back-and-forth, nauseating teeter-totter that I couldn't take any longer. He was there one minute, gone the next. Our marriage was so horrid that I couldn't keep up with how he felt about me any longer, and throwing people in the mix only made things worse. At one point he left me for another woman with my exact name, and I had started to date another guy named Christian. It was comical, but at the time, the things we did to get back at each other were so absurd that it was more exhausting to be apart than it was to be together. Vengeance was just as gratifying for me as prowling for sex was. He and I were so combative with one another that I had to take a page out of my parent's book on how to be vindictive to end our marriage. As if I hadn't already been.

I knew I wanted to end all contact with Christian, but it was hard to stand by my decision. No amount of sex or game-playing would help ease the pain from the love I felt. I was attached to him as if he were embroidered in my flesh. No one prepares you for the moment you get so locked in, from the tingle in your crotch to the first kiss, and the mesmerizing eye contact you make with meeting someone you know you want inside you. The feelings and sensations that evoke your spirit to come alive can be the very thing that tear you apart. I had very little control, as much as I was manipulating to get my way, I also was being manipulated. It was the lack of control I displayed around Christian that made me lose my mind. I wanted him as much as I didn't.

That madness pushed me over the edge and I wanted a reprieve from it all. My only solution was to cry out for help and what better way than to attempt suicide? Dramatic entrances and exits had always been a "go-to" of mine growing up, but suicidal thoughts weren't something I ever imagined sharing. I had had them on and off since I was 14, but couldn't articulate them with anybody, my parents included. I would write about how I would want to die and the details of my death in my journal, but never brought myself to act on it until one afternoon at my grandparents' mansion out in the country. It was when my aunt walked in on me naked in a bathtub with a bottle of pills tipped over ontop of the bathroom mat did she call for help. I swallowed a handful, enough to make me sick, not dead. I was hoping to be knocked out by the pills and drowned, but that didn't happen either. Turns out hormonal pills can't do that. Tragic for me at the time because that bottle would be the reason I got checked in at the Northwest Pavillion Hospital. Makes for a cavalier story to tell my bunkmate about how I ended up in such a mess over a person I loved. During the time I was with Christian, I had been in four other relationships, two female and two male, was forced to sell my car, lost my apartment, and had my first suicide attempt that landed me on the fast track for a psych evaluation. I'm pretty sure the lack of a thorough evaluation was why I was released, on top of my family vouching for me that I wasn't actually crazy or troubled. That it was no more than my dramatic antics at play. The second I was released I was ready to sign divorce paperwork so I could finaly have closure and move on with my life, but was forced to postpone filing them because Christain went A-wol and ended up in prison for years to come. We would stay married until I found him again 10 years later. I left Texas and ended up going back to where it all started. The place that I deemed to be the cornerstone of my downward spiral and trashy reputation. The place I thrashed myself around in as if I were some rag doll everyone wanted to play with. That place would be Fanta Se, New Mexico. This particular town was both disgustingly special and uniquely controversial. A place of many wandering young people, like myself, trying to find the nearest couch to crash on. In my case, a college dropout looking for the perfect relationship; it was a bed I was after. Screw your couch.

After a few weeks of being out, it was a kaleidoscope of body parts and feelings that led me to meet him. I hadn't wanted another Christian Mcall in my life, yet that would be the very template I would follow. A guy named Leo walked into my girlfriend's apartment with an "I've been dragged through the mud" demeanor and a pocket full of smokes when I quickly brushed him off. Why? My mind took me directly to what I always thought about pretty boys with long hair and soft features: you're gay. Man did I live in a box with how I perceived people. Maybe it was my ignorance, or how jaded I had been since I married a guy who liked guys, but I felt like I should have stayed away. With this in mind, I didn't give him a second look; why would I? I was already juggling a girl named Scarlette, who insisted that I spell her name "Skarlette" and a boy named Trevor. He went by multiple names so it didn't really matter what I called him. I could call this boy my sex toy and he would answer to it considering that he had a thing for doms, and he knew where he stood in our relationship: wherever I wanted him to. I had never been a dominatrix, but my attitude would suggest that I am the dominant one in relationships. Sometimes he and Skar would stand at the foot of the bed, waiting for me to tell them what I wanted next. Body surfing if you will.

They respected each other, but didn't love one another. I loved both, but didn't respect either. Yes, I know, the whole "how could you love without respect?" argument. It didn't matter to me that love may have included more than carnage. What I knew as love up until that point was all I had. Unfortunately, they were targets of my reckless passion for sex. My sex and the way I used it, performed it, and withheld it (I thought) was an amusing game they wanted to play. There was a reason they stuck it out. Being narcissistic wasn't enough to deter them from me, and I sure as hell liked to believe I was the best they'd ever had. I wasn't conscious at the time of how much power I really had over my lovers, but now that I look back… I am remorseful.

Skarlette took me into her studio apartment on the south side of town, since I had nowhere to go, fresh off the funny farm. I probably could have gone back to my family but I'm sure I would have ended up right back in the mental institution. So there I was, in the barrio with my white girlfriend, being reminded that if you don't speak Spanish, you'd better learn the head nod. It was my plump ass and fuck you attitude that made me welcome anywhere I went on the south side. I walked around like I had no fear. I thought that it was my face and my body that made people clear a path for me, and I was convinced it was my shield. The way others reacted to my presence made it acceptable - how could I be to blame?

I used my manipulation to win Skar over and became a house bunny for her. I couldn't really cook, so I tickled her interest with foul incentives. I couldn't bring in any money because I wasn't sure how, so I cleaned instead. Most importantly, I told lies to make believe a life she had always imagined living. My assumptions of what she could possibly want were so fucking wiley! I should have just asked her what she wanted out of the relationship, but that would require being selfless, so I thought it would be better to just stick to MY program. I was the trophy wife and she was the breadwinner. Some days when she was at work and I was home alone, I got a break and took off one of the many masks I wore to air out my long eyelashes. On those days, I would scheme on how to keep things going. It was a job in itself, so I guess you could say I did work. Skar provided me with things I needed to keep her going in my direction. A popcorn ceiling over my head, a car to run pointless missions in, food to keep my body full of hot air, and money for cigs and drugs to keep me fun! Alcohol was my favorite drug at the time. It was over liquor and weed one night at our place that I would meet Trevor.

Trevor Alejandro Sommers was a lover, fighter, and art extraordinaire. He signed TAS on everything around town and the graffiti world respected him. Alongside Skarlette and myself, Trevor was most enjoyable while elevated on drugs and sex. Though this individual was very talented, like most artists in town, you wouldn't catch him without a cig marked "Marlboro" hanging from his juicy lip, or his belt around his ankles with a female muse to follow. Trev and Skar had a lot in common. Pretty faces with parts of the body to match. And, a desire for me. What happens when three hot people have too much in common? No relationship could survive that much ego. They were constantly blaming one another for how they made the other the "odd man out". It was an oxymoron if you asked me. Pointing a finger, in our case, wasn't effective at all when we had originally claimed to be free and open to share each other. Turning around and stamping labels of limitations on who received love had me beyond confused. Some days Skar got me more than Trev did, and others, Trev got me when Skar wanted my attention.

I can appreciate rules and regulations within polyamorous relationships, such as not bringing back STDs or keeping the safety of each person involved by respecting their boundaries, but this - this was not a well-organized trio. It was the whole catch-22, agathokakological thing to me. How could love and hate exist so much in relationships? Do they just cancel each other out, love and hate? How could you love more than one person and jealousy not be involved? I was what they both shared, and I wasn't in a position to ask about their jealousy or insecurities when I was getting what I wanted. I wanted both and I wasn't going to accept anything less. Trevor didn't mind sharing me when he was sober; in fact, he would make jokes about how his girlfriend had a girlfriend. Having two lovers was standard for me. I did my best to keep it to just two lovers at one time. It was hard for me though…I couldn't help spinning a different web once I met someone else who wanted a piece of me. Monogamy was foreign to me and wasn't enough. Polyamory wasn't enough. Consent is usually on the table for all people involved, but I wasn't having that. I had already been addicted to being sneaky. How could anyone just want one person?

There was this one time Skarlette told me she cracked the bathroom door open to gasp for a clean breath (since she was going poop) and through the door's vertical slit she noticed me sitting on the couch with my belly hanging out over my spandex underwear, while my finger was stuck inside my belly button, eating a slice of Kraft cheese. String cheese was too expensive and you only got so many sticks in a package. I was playing with my belly ring while she was "admiring me" from afar. With her exhale she muttered, "I fucking love you." I was unaware that she was staring at me and when I finally looked up, her gentle voice grabbing my attention over the movie I had on as background noise, she said "I love you" again.

I smiled and couldn't help but say "I love you" back. The times I meant it were times like these. Vulnerable M.K. is the one that made people put up with her the other 90% of the time. It wasn't the loud, babbling drama that made them want me; it was brief exposure to my authentic, gentle self that helped them identify what they felt for me was real. There was also my rowdy sex; let's not forget that part. My sexual ability hooked them around the mouth, like a fish swimming upstream. Next thing you know, I gutted them and ate their fantasies with a spoon. It went great with my insecurities.

Greek mythology would suggest that a creature, a scaled woman perhaps, singing to lure away sailors is a siren— a prolonged noise, commonly to signal a warning. To me, a woman ensconced with mystery and a manner for sexual transactions fueled by lust is what they really mean. She drives herself toward a person(s) for a conquering, self-fulfilling prophecy. The goal of my siren... a reason to keep living. I was told by my sadistic stepdad, at 14 years old, that fear, vanity, and sex rule people's minds and are spoken languages for a siren. Neither Trevor nor Skarlette knew what they were in for by dating someone like me. Do I apologize for not sounding the alarm? Even if I felt my actions were justified by punishing them, I had no right to disregard their very human mistakes. I knew I felt like a mythical creature when I couldn't feel empathy like they did or acknowledge that I, myself, would make mistakes. I've heard it said that mercy is for those who show remorse, and I would force my lovers to beg me for my forgiveness. It seemed that I enjoyed the begging for my love and affection.

For instance, Trevor was a drunk and a junkie. I was too, but my delusion that I wasn't a junkie at the time, was more important. Typical behavior of an addict to gaslight the people they love the most. In a single night, I allowed myself to be shoved in a closet like some sex slave while being tossed around by Trevor. It was consensual, of course. I liked watching him have his way with me. Meanwhile, the house was bumping Bassnectar- Cozza Frenzy while partygoers walked right past the closest we were in with no clue of what was taking place. When Trevor and I got rowdy, it was nothing short of what I liked to call Porno Passion. Porno Passion is performative sex that entails a noticeable chemistry between two or more people, but the love is limited by the inauthentic acting. Fake orgasms or themed playfulness that doesn't necessarily show souls intertwining, but the passion for penetration. I knew Trev wasn't my forever person to have sex with, but I sure loved making him feel like he could be a runner-up. He was the first person that ever made me squirt! Who would have thought that female ejaculation could be so beautiful? Amen! Maybe amen isn't the right word for this celebratory moment, but you get the picture. I was obsessed with Trevor and he was obsessed with me.

This is also the guy who made me mount him in the closet while wearing Stilleto shoes as he grabbed each of my ass cheeks with his big, artistic hands to pull me into him as deep as he could go. He gripped me so tight and tugged me so eagerly I would reach my threshold as he pulled my cheeks apart from each other. A tear welled up in my eyes, I could feel blood trickling from my ass crack and I knew it couldn't have been cum since he was still thrusting. All I could think of was how this fucker would use my blood for paint if he could since he was that sick! What do I do? Do I tell him what he's done? This was a setup! My poor asshole. Of course, I sprang up off of him with my throbbing body screaming "OW!" He opened his eyes, though he couldn't see his own hand in front of him, and said with an out-of-breath tone, "What?!" I fell over to the side of him with my pants dangling around one ankle and had no response but to quickly scurry to the bathroom which was just a few steps away. I was so shocked and panicked, I could only imagine how he felt with a hard-on that would have no resolve by me. I pulled myself together long enough to shout for Skarlette through the crack of the bathroom door. What was it with that bathroom door being the ultimate means of communication around there! I clearly needed someone to assess the damage, since I couldn't just reach around and see for myself. After waiting what felt like too long, Skar finally responded to my screeching voice and I let out a sigh, knowing she wouldn't be prepared for this. I pulled her arm through the door and I could tell she was just as drunk as Trevor by how limber she was. The whole time I'm thinking, "Fuck! Why aren't I this lit[1]?" I told her what had happened and wanted her to fix it. All she could do initially was laugh. Who wouldn't? I looked over my shoulder, hunched over the toilet to pierce her with my eyes full of wrath. She shifted her laughter into problem-solving genius. She left for a few minutes only to return with a bottle of vodka and some Neosporin. She suggested a

---

[1] Lit = slang term my generation came up with for "High/Drunk"

band-aid, but how would that work? Anyway, after disinfecting my open wound, she kissed me and returned to the party, leaving me to deal with my blacked-out, drunk boyfriend.

Realizing that Trev could not comprehend what just happened because he was passed out cold on the floor near the bed, it was up to me to decide what my next move would be. It's too bad he made it out of the closet. I decided to try to wake him up to scorn him, but that didn't work. He must be punished. Even though it was an accident, he caused pain and embarrassment for me. That happens right? Asshole malfunctions? Only Skar and I knew what he did, so I could mold the night into whatever I wanted, misuse his mistake to get ahead in whatever sick game I was playing. I started with a scavenger hunt by leaving him a note in his pants that read, "You fucked up, it's over." So vague, but enough to get what I needed out of the situation…him to beg for me. If you asked me then why I did it, I would have told you because he deserved it. What he had done to my poor asshole was enough for me to act vengeful in the worst way. Psychological warfare was my shit. My M.O. if you will. What the fuck does "M.O." even mean? Typical me, using phrases I hadn't learned the meaning of yet. Not like I would let them know how cunning I was being, developing a skill to convince others of my bullshit. It's Modus Operandi (Latin, literally 'way of operating'), by the way.

Trevor woke up the next morning with a hangover and a scribbled note stuffed in his crotch and I recall purposely leaving the apartment early so he would wake up without me, wondering where I was. I let his bewilderment run for a while before I told him what happened. I enjoyed every minute of torturing him with all the gratifying power I knew I had, just waiting to get what I wanted. He was first conflicted, then sad since I suggested a breakup over this incident, and finally - he was sorry. Yes! I got him to apologize and extend offer upon offer before he knew the truth of what he did. I won. Simple as that. This was my tactic and I had no plan to stop. I was well on my way toward that Master Manipulator degree. Trev <u>Never</u> deserved that. He was the sweetest, most deep-kissing lover who exposed the depths of who he was to me at the time. He was interested in me, my thoughts and my body, and he always wanted to hold me tight every chance he got. He would paint me and make digital art that represented me in the most eye-catching way. It gave a whole new tone of flattery that I walked around with as my excuse for being "untouchable". Nobody could touch my unwavering attitude of egotistical gestures and even though Trev didn't think the punishment fit the crime, I wasn't about to relinquish my power over him.

Like I needed my head to be any bigger than it was, Trevor would always compliment me every chance he got. I'll never forget him being so impressed with how symmetrical my breasts were, and trusting his artistic vision, only added fuel to the fire. I needed to showcase those bad boys more often so why not try nude modeling? I couldn't help but explore my options the more my lovers hyped me up. This only bred more confidence in me to go out and capture someone else to replace Trevor. Between our movie-watching and music-humping, we always rolled together with danger lurking and living for the thrill of the moment. I was the model, he was the artist; it was perfect. It would seem that I had a routine for this sort of ritual. Mind you, he was the opposite of Skarlette. I loved the scale of this love triangle because Skar was my feminine and Trev was my masculine. Skar nestled me in her breasts and tickled my back while Trev spanked me and reminded me that I was not just pretty, but gorgeous. Why were these heads so important to me? It was the first love triangle I had ever been in. All my childhood insecurities would surface with them, and it was time to address the mommy and daddy issues that pushed me in their direction. But not before he walked through the door. We really needed to stop throwing parties so I could catch my breath.

Chapter 2

#Henoticesme#toobusydissapointing

It's still unclear how much time had gone by, but winter was approaching and I still hadn't come to terms with how unhealthy my behavior was. Not only was I exaggerating my victim mentality to get what I wanted, but I was abusing the shit out of my body. All I was longing for was the safety of my own home. I'm the proverbial, prodigal son (Luke 15:12). I wanted to go home, but I felt like I couldn't. I thought I was a sweetheart wrapped in my parents' healthy love, worthy of all the comfort and acceptance in the world, but really, I felt abandoned and misled so asking for anything was trumped by my shame. Throughout my childhood, I fought for attention and affection only to be faced with what I thought was my truth early on in life – that nothing I did would be good enough. After countless attempts to win people over, I found myself alone in spirit, and in mind. I was hungry for acceptance and desperate for attention. I needed to love and be loved. Kicking and screaming, I wanted to live in a world that understood what I wanted without explaining what it was I wanted. Between the smiling and the crying, I provoked people to question themselves when they were around me. I constantly questioned myself.

My addict brain thought that if I made people second guess themselves, then I could get a reaction worth holding on to. I lived for a visceral reaction. It took the attention off me for a brief moment so no one would notice how hurt I was. I didn't sit well when there were no elaborate emotions being shown, nor did I want to accept anything that wasn't fun for me, so I would search for comfort in what I deemed to be fun. Parties and people. Self-awareness was not my second language when I was partying. Neither was Spanish.

You know, my white-washed, Mexican lifestyle overshadowed the real roots of my culture and it couldn't have been more damaging, for me. It felt like my parents were ashamed of being Mexican to some extent, and so were their parents. I guess that's why I lied to Leo and told him I was Brazilian; he believed me by exaggerating a long look at my ass. All the slurs I had heard around Mexicans when I was a kid, and even now, had me trying to pass off as anything but. I'm an exotic-looking female and I knew that people assumed I spoke Spanish, or some other foreign language. I didn't. Not well enough to gain the respect of other Spanish speaking relatives. It wasn't until I realized how badly I wanted to fit into my own family that I learned to pay close attention when the OGs[1] were talking. Escaping to this country, my lineage was grateful for the landing, but naively hoping no one would notice how gutter they really were.

I noticed, and I loved it. They seemed to have resented it. I was told that my mother wasn't taught Spanish by my grandparents because they didn't want her to have an accent and get picked on in school. My father spoke fluent Spanish, but only if he knew it would benefit him directly. I spoke enough to pass off that I could be more

---

[1] Literally stands for "original gangster" but used to refer to someone with more experience/status

attractive, even cooler, if I understood what was being said when others couldn't. I chalked it up to me having to jump on the bandwagon of dissing my own culture since the guys I liked were as Anglo as it gets. Carla understood my culture; she was brown. Carla and I met when I was still with my first husband at a party I threw, of course. It was actually Christian who introduced me to Carla during our first semester at college. She put up with all of my antics and constant bullshit without complaining, so that pushed her up my rickety ladder into being a top-priority, best friend. She was beautiful. We'd flirted, but never touched. We'd kissed, but never sober. We'd argued, but never broke up for real, until we did. Carla took me to her tiny apartment once tension broke out in the Skarlette household.

So there I was, sitting on my friend Carla Hicky's couch, which would soon be my bed for a while, telling her my story of the trifecta breakup. It was an explosion of "Fuck yous!" I cried to her, explaining how the relationship with Skarlette and Trevor had unraveled. I was unphased by their hurt feelings, telling Carla how Skarlette walked in on me and so and so, on her bed, which led to a conversation on how disrespectful I was. Carla lit up a 6-foot bong, that I helped her bedazzle, and listened to my animated story. I explained how I had dropped hints to Skarlette that I wasn't fully interested in the relationship anymore when I stopped having sex with her. The only time we ever touched was when we were passing around our drunk bodies throughout the 200-square-foot apartment. Trevor and I naturally faded out when he noticed my attention was elsewhere. I continued to paint a splattered picture of what happened while Carla's bloodshot eyes gazed at me, insinuating she was really listening. I'm not sure she was fully invested since that bong rip had her flushed, but she leaned in enough for me to tell her how Skarlette invited a bunch of people over to celebrate my brother coming to town to visit me from Yellow, TX. My brother Jax and I are four years apart and we look like twins. I would always say that he is the male version of me.

Everyone and their bestie showed up to this mangled apartment for the festivities, even Trevor. Poor Trev received zero sympathy or attention from me after our breakup since I was too busy watching my baby brother like a hawk. As if I was justified in disregarding his fragile state. It was common for me to deflect and act as if nothing happened between us. Trevor who? I wanted to place my focus on Jax so I didn't have to talk to Trevor about the ins and outs of what happened between us. I wanted Jax to enjoy his time with me! Drinking… ok. Smoking… alright. No drugging! If I saw Jax headed to the bathroom with someone who wasn't a potential booty call, all hell was bound to break loose! I'll be damned if I catch my brother snorting lines off a bathroom sink! I spoke too soon with that booty call comment though, because that's exactly what he got. Some ass. Who he got it from makes for an epic headshake of disbelief. I stumbled through the dark with pathways of clothes and beer cans leading the way. I startled Skarlette and Jax when the shuffle prompted them to both stop pounding each other like rabid animals and look up at me. I quickly turned around and went to the kitchen to find Trevor to gossip with quicker than I could catch my breath. I did my best to keep my composure so, again, no one would see I was hurting. I wanted to scream! Trev was nowhere to be found so I went outside to smoke a cigarette in hopes of finding someone that would want to hear the news of such betrayal. My brother!? Gross. I had to tell someone about my very human feelings as tears formed. So much for being a mythical creature that's not susceptible to the pain of betrayal.

After walking in on my ex-girlfriend with my little brother, I knew moving in with Carla was the right decision at the time. Of course, I couldn't do much about Jax. He went back to Texas where he would be safe from my incessant nagging about hooking up with my ex; he knew his secret wouldn't leave that apartment because I was embarrassed. It's not like I could tell my mom or dad. As badly as I wanted to tattletail, I couldn't. I felt my revenge was settled just by leaving Skar where I found her - in that filthy apartment. I find it so sickening how quick I was to judge someone for what they did or didn't have when I had nothing at all. I was a tourist. I used everything everyone else had provided for me. I needed to look the part of a victim if Carla was going to take me in and be my saving grace.

Before I left Skarlette's apartment, Leo stopped by. The guy I had been ignoring— Leo Cooper. The chill guy with the pretty face I thought was gay, had been watching me all along. He was decent enough to listen to my troubles that night and I was grateful for how understanding he was with the whole "my brother was only 16 and slept with my ex" situation. How often can people really relate to their sibling sleeping with their exes? I'm dying to know. Leo knew just what to say and how to comfort me. He knew Skarlette and I were over, and before I had gotten all of my torn clothes out of her place, he stopped by to bring me a teddy bear to make me feel better. It wasn't just any teddy bear; it lit up and changed colors when you touched its fluffy paws. I loved it! I was taken aback by his gesture and dropped to my knees to cuddle the bear ever so tightly like a little girl wanting a hug. I looked up at Leo, holding back tears, and thanked him for my raver teddy bear that lit up the room as bright as my bubblegum pink hair.

Leo came down to my level, and stared me in the eyes, and said, "Of course M.K., I got you." I hadn't ever heard my name said so gently that the whole world seemed to stop at the sound of it. That's when it happened. He leaned in to kiss me and life stood still for a brief moment. I should have told Carla about Leo when I was sharing my break-up diaries with her, but I didn't. I left that part out, knowing that Leo being in the mix would change everything.

After being at Carla's house for a month, I got a chance to listen to her life story and get out of my own problems for a split second. It was then I discovered amongst all her overly-ripe gossip that she and Leo had a thing going on at that time, and how Skarlette had given him a blowjob before I started dating her. Great, I'm attracted to a guy that my ex has sucked off and my bestie is talking to. I wanted to be sly and drop nuggets of info about how I was attracted to him, and I may have kissed him, but I didn't mention our kiss at any point. I failed to mention Leo altogether on purpose, first and foremost because she flagged Leo as a creep who kept trying to hook up with her after she directly told him she didn't want to. She clearly liked keeping him around. I guess she was trying to take things slow?? Taking romantic relationships slow was something she only did sober. That's how Carla worked. She liked the idea of being front and center, being a pussy queen, but couldn't bring herself to sit on the throne. I get it. I practiced this very tactic when I was a rug-rat. Now that I was no longer prepubescent, it was time to pounce. If I saw it, and wanted it, I got it. She was always a closet slut; instead of letting her freak-flag fly, she would spill secrets about her little black book to those of us that made fun of her for acting prude, knowing she wasn't. Since I was an out-in-the-open slut, I didn't understand why Carla couldn't make up her mind about Leo. I'd soon help her.

I hadn't talked to Leo after he kissed me, mainly because we never swapped numbers - just saliva. He was mysterious. Where was he? I thought about it from time to time but couldn't really bring myself to hunt him down with all that I had going on. My feelings of conquering him as some conquest weren't strong enough. My busy schedule of hooking up with random people I found out-and-about was more of a priority. Anyone outside of my friend circle was doable. I really didn't want to be with someone who could compare how having sex was with me versus with my friends. This is how I coped with losing love. Lustful moments were a cure-all for me. I needed to take my power back to feel desirable and not used up. Fresh meat would do the trick.

There was this one instance when I was leaving the mall and some guy in a nice car rolled his window down and asked me if I needed a ride. I didn't have a car at the time and he was hot. I politely, in a teasing manner, told the guy that I don't get cars with strangers and his disarming giggle had me hooked. Geez, it really didn't take much for me. He looked my age. I never felt a threat or danger around men because most of the time I felt like their puppeteer. I exuded an attitude of "I'll bite your dick off if you try me in any way," and it was intimidating to most. Even though I was taught by my father to never talk to strangers, let alone have sex with them, I wanted to find out how it felt to shave against the grain. My dad wanted me safe, but I wanted to gamble. I acted invincible, cocky, and had been taught how to fight, so I put myself anywhere I wanted. I had this guy, whose name I don't remember, take me to Carla's, posing it as my own place since she wasn't home. I had my panties dropped to my ankles and my body bent over the edge of her bed. He was sexy with every sound and hair tug. Something so brief ended with me telling him to leave immediately after we were done, giving me the high I needed. Carla came home and I was as innocent as an ant roaming on the kitchen counter looking for sugar. It was as if nothing had happened and my sleezy secret of anonymous sex was no big deal.

Over some ganja and beer, as per usual, Carla had proposed a trip to a town 45 minutes away from where we lived for a party for the night. I had already had my fix, so I was cleared for take-off. I wanted to share with her my craving for promiscuous fun over the road trip, but it seemed like an opportunity to slip up and say something to get me kicked out. I could reminisce with her about the time we went to Colorado for a rave where I almost died from taking a triple-stacked ecstasy pill. But why the hell would I bring that up? Who really wants to relive the time you overdosed on a "feel good" drug? I still get creeped out at the thought of convulsing and my eyes rolling into the back of my head, but smile when I think of the guy who saved me. I owe that stranger my life. So, small talk it is! I was sure Carla would settle for small talk and as I geared up to open my mouth, she told me we were going to party with none other than, Leo.

"Leo Cooper?" I asked. She said we were going in his car and spending his money to get there. I agreed hesitantly. I guess we were doing this. Why the hell not? I was already keeping a secret about my mid-day rendezvous, so in my mind, I thought it was going to be fun, collecting more obscene secrets. Amongst the awkward fact of Leo and I sharing a kiss, which we both were handling remarkably well I might add, he was surprised to see me again under the pretense of a party trip with Carla, his love interest. I was thinking about how scandalous the night was going to turn out to be. So many twists and turns. I was getting used to this web of attraction.

All night Carla and Leo portrayed behavior of being "just friends". I was baffled. It would be later that Leo and I found ourselves alone to chit-chat over how I was fucking one of his best friends while I was living with Skarlette. "You know, so and so?" His name was Adam. He was the one Skarlette took revenge over. I was a busy girl. Adam was

Leo's best friend; my brief sideline pleasure. It was only one time, and Skar had interrupted so it wasn't like I would count it. It was a few thrusts before we had to jump off each other. He was fun while it lasted, but no big deal to me. I immediately noticed Leo was jealous that his friend had been inside of me and he was just NOW meeting me. I couldn't help but let him know how I knew about the Skarlette blowjob thing and hinted to him that I don't play with guys that have been with my exes. My honesty always came out as bragging. Though I was admitting our mutual friendships, like Skar and Adam, I also had a boastful tone regarding my sexual interactions, especially if the person I was talking about knew them. Leo left our conversation that night puzzled about what to do next. Pursue me, or leave me be? The night ended and the party continued in my head as we made our way back home. Leo's appearance grew seemingly sexier the more I observed him. Us girls were safely home, the three of us locked eyes, said goodnight, and Leo was on his way. I walked inside the house and thought, "Is this my second go at a threesome? Carla and Leo? Could they possibly be my next love triangle?" I passed out drunk on the couch to see what my answers would be in the morning.

It had been two months of living with Carla as a free-spirited bum slut. No car. No job. Just pussy and a pretty face to float my mooching ass on by. I was merely surviving using my goods; is that so bad? I felt liberated by my body count, yet I was tossing away my life by doing nothing but partying and fucking. It seemed to be more than appropriate to fill the void. I wanted direction, but who would give it to me? I needed a project, but what would it be? Carla's cousin Cameron stopped by for a visit and I knew instantly that he was my next project. Damn, the doors that let attractive people in. He was a tough one to narrow in on. Cameron was a motocross-riding country boy with the prettiest smile I had seen in the last 48 hours. Most importantly, Cameron was a challenge. He had just gotten out of a relationship, and he showed the slightest interest in having a rebound. Challenge accepted. As I spent our party nights at the house getting to know him and seeing pictures of his ex, I got a chance to do some recon to make him mine. My methods were absurd, I know…but before Cameron saw me again… I'd be ready. It took no more than a day to give myself a makeover to woo Cameron into my world. My sexual world of manipulating people into what they think they want, exposing their sexual desires, instead of letting them decide for themselves. Or maybe, they really did know better and still wanted to mess with me; either way, it gave me purpose. I was ready to make Cameron realize his broken heart was nothing to fret over.

I woke up the next morning after all the premeditative flirting and went to the bathroom with a pair of scissors to cut my hair. It was still very pink and his ex-girlfriend was a brunette, which I naturally was, but he didn't know that. Her hair was short too so I gave myself a swing bob. Short in the back and long in the front, right under my chin. I took a shower and scraped change to go buy some cheap, box of hair dye to make my hair pitch black. I threw on one of Carla's FOX riding T-shirts and a pair of jeans as if I were some muddy, motocross-riding chick. I had ridden 4-wheelers before but never a dirt bike. Who would know, right? I'm a chameleon. I normally dress spunky and loud, never been a plain T-shirt and jeans girl, but hey… I looked good and, most importantly, I played the part even better. He was coming over soon and I had to be ready. Nightfall had shown up before he did, and it felt ominous outside. My new look was not to go unnoticed. He walked through the door and saw me first amongst the crowd of people shoved in that tiny duplex. Once we looked at each other, I felt a strong sensation in my stomach. I could give him a chance to run, I told myself. He had this look in his eyes that asked me to fuck him in the most polite way, to be gentle with his heart. I couldn't help myself even if I wanted to. Cameron Holt… you are mine for the night.

Booze flowing and couch sex under a blanket ended the night since we were the last two standing. Everyone was gone or passed out cold, and we had the chance to get sweaty. I rode Cameron in such a sensual way he had no words other than, "Can we do this again?" I said yes. We became a thing after that night for a couple of weeks. Most of the rebound, pseudo-relationships I started lasted no more than a month. Non-stop sex and whispers of sweet nothings into each other's ears, anywhere and everywhere we could. All the others were obsolete when I was using, including Leo. If you've ever seen a person take a drag from a cigarette, noticing the deep inhale they search for, you watch as whatever was plaguing them goes away—for a moment. They keep dragging the cigarette for reassurance that they can escape the situation and feel the rush instead. The exhales of smoke leaves their mouth and those of us watching either judge in disgust, or relate to the lightheadedness. Cameron was my inhale. Letting him go was my exhale. Like most cigarette butts, you flick them and never think twice.

I put in effort to make Cameron forget his girlfriend long enough to entertain me and my sexual cravings. He was great. He would be my first exploration of shape-shifting for love. How can I taper myself to get the guy? Or girl? Cameron eventually had to go back to his small, shit-kicking town a few hours away and I was able to go back to being me. Who was that exactly? A transition from character to character became a habit for me. Who will I be next? Sick! Right? No, seriously, I got sick so I had no other choice other than to go home to my dad's house to let him take care of me. I was a stubborn, ill woman. Still thinking I could be with my drug-induced friends and heal my poor fragile body was not an option. That's exactly what I was: fragile. My heart was brittle to the touch and the way I cared for my body was with alcohol and sex. When push came to shove I was down and out, and I was sure I could never overstay my welcome with my friends, but I would soon find out that that wasn't true with my father.

Chapter 3

#Daddyissues#familytree#uprooted

I showed up at my dad's house two days before Christmas, looking as sorry as ever. I was trashed from partying, sore from all my foul play, and I had a fever which caused snot to drip down to my swollen lips. I wiped my nose with my sleeve as my dad answered the door. I go inside his beautifully remodeled home to be greeted by Christmas decor imitating a storybook, reminding me of how innocent I once was. I really wanted to rest, eat, and be pampered by Daddy; however, what I got was my dad locking up the medicine cabinet and a few words grunted here and there. I could tell he was annoyed. I thought surely my dad, out of all people, would be there for me in my time of need since it was routine for him to remedy my situation. I walked out of the kitchen after feeding myself and noticed what I really wanted was to be fed nurturing care. I wanted medicine for my cold, but all I got were cold gestures. What was happening? Was he mad at me?

My father's stern voice snapped at me when I was lying on the couch half coherent. "M.K., I don't want you in my room looking for medicine. They're controlled substances and I don't trust you with them." I'll never forget the feeling I had, aside from congestion from the head cold, when my father said he didn't trust me. Had I been that far gone to the point that my dad didn't trust me with antibiotics? I wasn't even thinking about abusing pharmaceuticals. You know, stealing from your parents' medicine cabinet to sell or consume is pretty common, apparently, but I was just trying to feel better. It was then and there that I felt sorry for myself, enough for that pang in my heart to make me feel alone and scared. Daddy's little girl was not being treated like his princess, instead like a villain. I had burned my daddy's girl bridge, ladies and gentlemen.

I'm sure it had happened sooner, I just didn't notice the flames consuming our relationship before. I remember crying like I was 13 all over again, having to meet my new stepmom for the first time as I lay on the couch and watched him lock himself in his office. I just wanted my dad to care for me since I was sick, but it was being sick in more than one way that pushed him to draw a line in the sand. My dad had seen such inconsistency with my behavior that it was no wonder he would want to take the necessary precautions. I had used and abused my title of "daddy's girl" as an adult and it wasn't cute anymore. All the get-out-jail-free cards I played because of who he was started to grow stale.

Every lawyer I needed for breaking the law and every ticket scratched off with the knowledge of my last name had added to my untouchable behavior. "Do you know who I am? My dad will have your balls on a platter officer (blah blah blah) if you don't let me go!" I'm sure the embarrassment my dad felt had taken up more real estate than not. I was treated as suspicious for good reason. He knew I was throwing parties at his house and still let me live in his garage. He knew I was tormenting him to get back at him, yet he still wanted me around. Until he didn't. When I came to him in the shape I was in, he knew something was up and he let me know he could NOT stand by it any longer.

My dad had cut me off once when I was 14 and for two years I didn't get any "happy birthdays" or phone calls reminding me that I was loved by him, only to later find out it was because I had told him that I thought my stepdad was a better father than he was, on top of other reasons I'm sure. And just like that, my dad was absent and letting me know his silence was saying something his words couldn't. He used to give my mom the silent treatment, and I can see where it drove her mad. It's damaging. I've ghosted people before and I do believe it is a torturous act, no matter the intention behind it. It wasn't until I was 16 that I got an email from him with a song by *Stainded* called *Sweet Zoe Jane* attached to it, expressing his feelings about not being around. I knew he missed me but not having my dad in my life pushed me to accept that it would be a thing for us. Periods of time without speaking and then coming back together to catch up and love each other, as if nothing happened.

Each time we reunited, I would learn some truth about why he abandoned me and did my best to stomach his trauma dumping before I ever had a chance to tell him about myself. I'm not shaming him, he has every right to have a dark past and mistakes so deep that most wouldn't forgive, but I didn't know how to show grace towards him at the time. All I wanted was to love and hate him at the same time. I made decisions that revolved around him and wanted to make him feel better over my own feelings and boundaries. This kind of dysfunction in our relationship had me living in fear of disappointing or losing him again, so I would swallow the harsh truth about what he thought of me, and i never challenged his words or feelings. I would walk away more brokenhearted each time he shared his truth. I had my own truth, but never brought myself to share it with him until I sobered up.

After I woke up from a NyQuil-induced nap, I knew it was time to leave and find a place of my own since I had been sleeping on Carla's couch. I needed somewhere to live and have some independence. My dad was always available to help me out financially, which was frequent when I was using, but I never really helped myself with what was given. Ever heard of that saying "never give an addict money?" I wanted my dad to respect me, love me, and support me but I wasn't sure how to do any of that without my own self-respect. I constantly felt the urge to fill the void of my dad with other men but failed to know that it was just my own "Daddy issues" preventing me from hopping off the hamster wheel. What are "Daddy issues?" Let's talk about them...

My parents were the specimens of a sheltered line of parenting, and saying that they each had it rough growing up would be a colossal understatement. Their parents and their parents' parents trickled a special type of generational mess. Aside from being taught to survive the cruelness of society for being Mexican, they learned to stay tight-knit with each other and didn't socialize much outside of their clique. We could easily place blame on the complexities of my family's teachings, but instead, we will just say it resulted in very shut-down parents which, in turn, led to a shattered parenting style. If I blame them now, I would just be perpetuating the systemic trauma; but before I excuse them, I'm here to pinpoint how I was affected by their decisions directly. I learned early on that my parents weren't confident in each other so the way they were parenting was split in two, causing confusion for everyone. Cultural standards and traditions mixed with disagreeing and undermining each other made for some turbulent times in our household. My parents always struggled with being on the same page, and it showed. I didn't mind if my parents' stories lined up since I was governing myself most of my tween years. It was whether or not I would take what they said into consideration that helped me decide who I wanted to be more like.

My dad led with an iron fist while my mom would cower and slip into a distracted state that seemed to have pulled her in a thousand different directions. My rebellious behavior took hold the moment I discovered I could use their parenting styles against them. I'm sure you've heard that saying "DO AS I SAY AND NOT AS I DO," implying that the behavior displayed shouldn't be copied but to trust the words that were said as if they held some sort of merit. Well, I never really cared to respect them at all because of how unbalanced their behavior was. I wanted them to lead by example but it seemed that that wasn't on the table with how inconsistent things were. I'm sure they tried but it wasn't sticking. It wasn't until I was long gone, living my own life, that I noticed they were evolving into people who respected their word. Part of the example they were trying to set was through religion when there were so many pseudo-Christians in the church, but witnessing my parents' attempt to lead by faith was something I knew they wanted for us kids. I remember going to church with them both before they split and not really feeling the impact because I was too young.

It wasn't until they remarried that Church became somewhere I dreaded going since I blamed everyone and the world around me for why my parents divorced. I had a hell of a time trying to assimilate, and the resentment began to build. There was this one time I was felt up by a boy named Mitch during a weekday church camp I attended, and I didn't know what to do other than stay quiet about it. That same church was also a school that would soon struggle with a scandal blasted all over town about a teacher sleeping with one of her students. All I could do was shake my head and ask myself "What's the point?" The corruption was in my home and the church, so why bother? I couldn't find solace anywhere and although I could appreciate the attempts to have us three children grow up around a church environment, it just wasn't effective for me no matter how many times we said grace around the dinner table. If anything, it turned me away from it in the worst way. I hated the thought of the church until later in life when I grew a better understanding of what my parents were trying to accomplish.

I was able to identify from an early age how caring, hardworking, money-hungry, and title-savvy my parents were. Even though there was this glimmer in my eye that my parents could do no wrong, I knew something was amiss. I can't pin them too hard for wanting to build a fruitful environment for their firstborn. It wasn't ALL bad. Being the oldest child and only girl, for a while, had its perks. My dad was the first to hold me when I arrived at BSA Hospital on October 18, 1990. Some experts say that the first parent who holds you at birth will be the one you connect with most. It would seem that he stepped in to cradle me while my mom had to be rushed to the operating room for life-saving surgery. I was next to be ripped from his arms since I almost died that day, too. My harsh entrance to this world can be taken into account as a start for all the trauma I was about to experience. I'm not above certain theories, but I also don't think that my survival was in vain. My dad held me and just like that, he was my first love connection.

I will say that I am connected to both my parents on an even playing field now, but that was my choice, not theirs. Back then, I would go back and forth trying to decide which parent I favored most, and as I grew up, I realized the importance of having a healthy relationship with them both; leaving nepotism out of it, even if they didn't know what it meant to have a healthy relationship. I was still learning what it meant to have healthy tendencies and boundaries but that was because I chose to keep up with the times while they were struggling with what it meant to be progressive with their communication styles. I credit them for their journey through therapy and learning about themselves, but none of that was present when I was under their roof.

Sometimes the child has to be the parent and after years of wanting my family to communicate in a way that was productive and effective, I knew it was time to be part of the movement I so desperately wanted. Part of doing that was first loving and forgiving my parents for faults that added to my distress. Then, it was accepting them for who they were/are so I could start to live my life freely without the burden of the past. What else was I left to do with two parents that were taught to be quiet? I wasn't very good at being quiet and it would sometimes result in being told by my parents that I was ALL my mother or ALL my father regarding my behavior. In reality, I was a balance of them both with perfect destruction and production. I didn't know the effect my words would have on my life until I was ready to be loud for the right reasons. But before that took place, my active addiction took control and ran rampant, playing my parents' faults against them. It was how I was able to punish them for the paths they dragged me on. I didn't believe the power of my tongue could bring life or death (Proverbs 18:21), and I would learn that lesson when the very thing I did to them was being done to me.

Lars Alanzo Reyes was the epitome of rags to riches, "fire in my belly, never going to let my kids go without," father. A hard-up Mexican boy from the hell pits of Juarez, he took on the world at a young age. Born into danger, and growing up in danger, it seemed like the danger never left him. It's no wonder he chose an adrenaline-pinching career and couldn't sit still unless he napped himself into submission. The man has been conditioned. I remember him teaching us kids how to make sandals out of newspaper not knowing at the time that he was just giving a hands-on example of how he survived. I thought it was the coolest thing to walk around my two-story house with hand-made chanclas. I looked at all the effort he put into giving us everything that he didn't have as no big deal. His crying was the big deal. Isn't that the way? Trauma embedded into your brain, that deep, can only motivate you to do something to ease your mind and heart.

My mother, Kristi Lee Reyes, was the red lipstick mark of beauty, and Lars was an authoritarian figure to the public eye and a looker I might add. Both of them. My friends always reminded me how hot my parents were and never let me live it down. I hated having attractive parents. My father really is a brilliant mind, but he suffered from a lack of emotional connection with my brothers and me. It's odd because I saw him and my mom being affectionate with one another, even romantic at times. She was always scratching his back while he laid in her lap on the couch, or there was this one time he planned a scavenger hunt for her birthday and I thought it was the sweetest thing to the point where I ended up duplicating that very scavenger hunt for some of my lovers. My mom was beautiful. It was no wonder she participated in beauty pageants when she was a teen and caught the eye of my father.

My parents met on the swim team in high school and it was definitely puppy love turned obsession. Their love had been unhealthy to a colossal degree, in my opinion, and after each parent stated their case of how things went down between them, I ultimately landed on confirming they were meant for each other, but that's neither here nor there. It's a shame they didn't stay together because I do believe the two of them shared beautiful moments that could have lasted if they hadn't been so young and stubborn. Oh, and there is always how neglectful they were towards their mental health. It wasn't a concept they were taught about, so why would they address their psychosis? My mom had me right after she graduated high school and the pressure to marry each other was strong. Trauma breeding trauma. I was born into an unhealthy love and I gave birth to a child from unhealthy love. I'm grateful my big, Mexican family was around to help while my parents did their best to figure things out, but whatever they were doing wasn't working. It felt as if I was doomed from the get-go after learning each horrid story of the mischief they caused like cheating on each other and kidnapping me from the other; it was apparent that the maturity was in low supply. If it were a game of chess, I was definitely the pawn.

It takes a village to raise children, I'm told, and my village helped tinder a fire of hope that things could be ok for me in life and I could have a chance to become whatever it was I aspired to be. I believe it takes a village to support a mother and even though part of my reality was being looked at as nothing more than a statistic, I had hope. When you realize that embracing the culture you were born into by being a proud, Mexican girl isn't an option, you just condition yourself to be something else. As I began to comprehend my home life, I knew my attempts to fit in were a misfire. I knew my family had escaped to the States for a better life but the disguises they wore to go under the radar would affect generations to come. I didn't speak Spanish fluently and I embraced white culture more than my own. I felt the need to keep the facade going with all they went through, so denying my ethnicity was just the beginning. I pulled the "I'm European, Asian, Islander, and Russian" thing at least once or twice in my life. I was always identifying as American/White before Mexican because I realized how it gave me status. I was looked at with respect if I claimed the American part of my identity before the Mexican.

Oh, the American way. The dichotomy of profiling and inclusion is real. Always selling the idea of dreams and aspirations for anyone to attain as long as you know a guy, who knows a guy, and that guy knows he's white. My family was oppressed, and when you throw some "American Dream" on top of it, it caused vivid images of the sacrifices they made just so we could be trusted and not looked at as anything more than wet-backs. I saw the chip on my father's shoulder, so why not have one myself? My mother was raised to not go outside her home, ever, and that her family was all she needed. Talk about socially awkward. That explains a lot about why I am one of two ways– extremely introverted or extremely extroverted. It was fear that kept my lineage so close to one another. Too close, I would say. That kind of environment had a ripple effect on us kids as we grew older and the only way I could break free from such enclosed thinking was to travel. Pretending to be someone everyone would like and accept seemed like something I could do. Until I took the acting role too far.

Kristi and Lars spent years tormenting each other, bowing down to each other's needs all-the-while planting seeds of insecurity that later would be taken out on us kids. It was over the course of their 10-year marriage that they became spiritually bankrupt and were hurting each other more than loving each other. I credit them for trying to keep the family together, but it wasn't something they felt they could accomplish anymore. They both grew bitter over those years and it only got worse after they divorced. I was constantly treating my mom and dad as if they were small children in desperate need of a hug once I learned each of their truths about the past. I wasn't always patient with them, mind you. I did pick up their learned behavior of torment, but my goal was to always have them in my life. Maybe it was their childhood trauma that kept them both in a chokehold, preventing healthy communication with me, or maybe it was the lack of self-worth that took them down such a windy road, who knows? What I do know is that they both had good and bad ways of loving me.

The love my mom showed me could be twisted and guilt-tripping, but she got better with each comment on how I could perform more to her standard. Kristi never failed to show up on the frontlines of battle with me no matter what kind of jam I got myself into. And my dad shows me love with his words, now, better than ever, even though he still goes on anger binges. I believe things will get better. I have to believe things will look up even though the same man who brought me the tenacious attitude to chase my dreams is the very person who abandoned me when I was nine years old and continued to do so up until recently. I still chose to love him through it all. That's one benefit of being a love addict; you never want to stop loving no matter how unhealthy things can get.

Finding a glamor shot photo of the woman my dad cheated on my mom with, in his coat pocket, was the nail in the coffin to my first round of daddy issues. After my mom examined the evidence I brought her, I watched my father throw a black trash bag full of his bad choices over his shoulder and head for the door. I'm sure there were plenty of reasons my parents called it quits; however, I was made to believe I was the reason. Talk about a heavy burden. I was innocent and my parents knew the truth, but no one told me. I would walk through life for years thinking I was at fault. The weight of the divorce set on my shoulders no differently than all my dad's belongings over his. He was the adult and I was the child; why would I have to endure that guilt when I should have been reassured that I wasn't the problem? I gathered all my markers and crayons to draw him a picture that day, to say I was sorry, and when I went to hand it to him before he left, he looked at me with eyes of despair and threw it away. That moment would be the first of many shameful feelings to jumpstart my addiction.

Even though my parents were divorced, money wasn't an issue (to my knowledge anyway) with every need being met and then some. My father had a legal profession that provided fair ground to play on and my mother worked many different jobs before getting her hands in the Insurance business. She also had my oil-rich grandparents to turn to when shit got complicated. After Lars moved out of the house and took his indignant attitude with him, it was a race to see who would remarry first. Everyone has an opinion on how this played out between my parents, but what matters is what I thought, felt, and experienced. This was my POV[1].

My mother had been through a few men before she landed on Andy Gonzalez. After exploring the dating realm, Kritsti ended up marrying Andy when I was 12, which everyone was a bit shocked about solely because she hadn't known him very long. I get it, three kids and needing some provision from a man, a new household leader, but that didn't mean it was the greatest choice for us kids. My dad still wasn't remarried to the woman he had been cheating on my mom with. Maybe because he knew, deep down, my mom still had his heart. I remember him taking me on dates with Patty (that's her name) while he was still with my mom. How could I forget those green eyes, stubby nose, and permed blonde hair? That woman was the black, poisoned apple in my fairy tale and I was coaxed into taking a bite. Sharing my dad with Patty left such a bad taste in my mouth, and I knew the moment she came into existence that I was going to have to fight to survive in my dad's life.

---

[1] POV = point of view

Shortly after the torch was lit by my mom, it was passed to my father. He ended up marrying Patty when I was 13. What an age to be hurled through forceful acceptance. I will never understand my parents. What were their motives for the decisions they made back then? No one will ever know but them. I can take a wild guess; an educated, Psych 101 evaluation of what they were trying to accomplish, but still, it wouldn't matter. Even if I had the answer, the damage was done. A lot of my focus was on my baby brothers, Blake and Jax. At least I was old enough to know some of the important details of what was going on unlike them. As time passed with my two, new families molding together, it was getting harder to keep up. I couldn't get on board with how my parents were living with their (supposed) significant others. I didn't know at the time, but their marriages would eventually rot out after a series of hapless events.

I took pride in my creative exploration of manipulating my parents. To play people to get what I wanted, or to avoid getting what was unwanted, required a bold attitude and some truth-bending. Once I began to flirt with the malevolent skill of pitting them against each other, I refined my practices to use in other areas of life. It was all the double birthdays and the constant barrages of "I'll just go ask Mom!" that gave me a fierce fighter in my corner. Neither parent liked feeling inferior to the other, and I picked up on that quickly. My father's house had the disciplinary structure of military-style living. Rooms were pre-designed barracks and the consequences included routine exercising and educational boredom, with the occasional door off the hinge. That was super unhealthy, in retrospect, for a young girl. The struggle to be heard and understood by my dad was real. No matter how I tried to get his attention, he was always occupied with something and his time was short. Sure, happy memories of adventurous vacations and gifts were always there, but the ability to parent me with the amount of attention I needed wasn't. His inability to be present was noticeable and even though he would hug and kiss me, I hardly witnessed the emotional intelligence from him when it came to helping identify my feelings as a young girl.

The man worked any chance he got, even if it was around the house. A true craftsman, and he is as impressive with his positive attributes as he is with his negative. I used to hype my dad up so often that I would later have to break down the standards I set for him as my hero, learning he is merely human. What a shattering realization that was. When I was at my dad's house, I noticed his priorities were building things to be bigger and better, including his family, but it seemed that things would constantly come unraveled at the seams. It would later cause my resentment towards him. The man's accolades are many and his resume speaks for itself, but I didn't gather his hard work as a direct connection for relationship building. His priorities were clear from his actions and I was too young to understand why I felt left out. I understand that I made my own decisions later on to push my dad away, so he had no say about feeding me any spiritual guidance or learning about me individually, but even if I hadn't, would he make himself available to do those things? He was always talking about how hard he had it growing up, and the crooks in his life helped motivate him into becoming an upstanding police officer. I'll always love him for that but he placed his career over undivided attention for his kids. Starting out as a corrections officer, then a police officer working the graveyard shift, my dad followed his calling and did the best he could. I know that. I remember him bringing donut holes for me and my brothers when he would get home as we were just waking up for the day. Those donut holes gave me reassurance that he didn't die on duty.

I was old enough to worry about my daddy not coming home. It caused panic attacks, but I didn't know what those were at the time. My dad eventually became a detective working in the Crimes Against Children Division which meant he underwent more stress. Being a good cop at the expense of his mental health was scary to watch, no different than him watching me succumb to addiction I'm sure, except I wasn't helping people.

He didn't stop at detective: undercover narcotics agent, S.W.A.T. medic, spokesman, and finally retiring with the status of chief. But let's be real, he never really quit working. Him and I are actively working towards better living and I was able to make amends with him after my epiphany of him being just another human being, like me who was hurting on the inside. Ever hear the saying, "hurt people, hurt people"? Well, Lars had his hurt leak into our household like toxic gas, waiting for the spark to blow the place up. Instead of our home catching the explosion, it was my heart and mind that disintegrated with all the hurt that was perpetuated. Being with my dad meant I fought for attention in the worst way with Patty as my stepmother. As a teenage girl, this was not the best way to prepare me for my adult years. I was left under her watch when my dad wasn't around, and she would torture me on purpose by singling me out and talking bad about me in front of other people. She once told my dad that she thought I was going to kill her in her sleep. That was the kind of melodrama that ruled the household, not to say I didn't add to the mix, but I was the child, not the adult. I was constantly left to shut down and was insecure about being in my dad's life.

Even though Patty was intolerable, I remembered my dad doing his best to instill memories of togetherness. Lord knows he tried sometimes but nothing he did was going to make me like her. Aside from the slue of women I had to fight for my dad's attention, the good times also stuck. There were nights we would gather in the hot tub and talk about life. He would ask us how our days went and what our highlights were, and I loved him for that, but never mind talking about how desperate we were to express our feelings because it was a no-cry zone with him. We were kids who had big emotions and were always afraid to express them. It was hard to gauge when it was an appropriate time to be a vulnerable kid around my dad or if we needed to suck it up and move on.

My dad couldn't involve himself in our lives without having to overcompensate later. He would grow angry and then make up for it with something that would pique our interest. Usually something fun. But what fun was it to actively be in a custody battle with my mom over us? The scales of happiness and sadness were constantly being tipped and I saw the confusion for Blake and Jax when a Forensic Psychologist bombarded us with questions we didn't understand. My mom wasn't going down without a fight and I felt compelled to take care of my brothers and be their voice. This was one of the areas I felt forced to grow up too fast in. The divorce was mostly a custody battle that turned into a pissing contest. Kristi was forking over money for the fight and Lars had the connections in the department. At what point was it about us and our well-being and not about who was going to win? Maybe in their mind they were fighting for our well-being by trying to keep us for themselves? That's not what happened for me. Not knowing how closely I was watching, my attitude of always being right and wanting to have the last word would soon hatch by watching my parents duke it out.

Truth be told, I didn't want to live with either of my parents or their lovers. I believe both my parents are love addicts and I am a product of that. My issues with wanting my dad's unconditional love from a young age up until now have helped me identify why I jumped from relationship to relationship, chasing something that wasn't there. What I needed out of my dad was the very thing I ended up giving myself, and I now see that my expectations for my dad in the past vs now are without parallel. He can't give away something he doesn't have. I forgive him, and the child in me that he hurt has been healing every day. Lars was an enigma in my eyes. He was warm and kind but also harsh and vulgar. Romantic and charming, yet womanizing and misogynistic. Handsome with a disarming presence, and once he was vulnerable, people opened up and told him the truth. His appearance wasn't just intimidating because he wore a badge, but his stature and tattoos would imply how strong he was. He would show his soft side through his passions, and teaching me was one of his passions. He loves being useful and constantly educates himself. He is a walking encyclopedia and taught me to measure twice and cut once. I didn't particularly care for it then, but I ate it up. I was told by an old boyfriend that my brain was too big for my britches and Lars is a huge reason why.

It was the lessons that he didn't directly teach me that I also took notes on and those were the lessons I would have to unteach myself, but not before I caused a ruckus. It would take years before I undo the damage of my upbringing with my dad. It's been documented by the Children's Bureau of Southern California that young women who have healthy relationships with their fathers are less likely to be clinically diagnosed with mental illnesses such as depression or anxiety. To me, the father-daughter relationship is of the utmost importance for the healthiness of the daughter, and I had to make the conscious decision that was what I wanted moving forward. I credit myself for my health level today, and if there is anything being self-made has taught me, it was that I can take back ownership of my life and what I want for it. My parents did what they knew how to do and I'll always love them. The effort they show today is like none other I've seen in my life. Just like I'm growing, they are growing alongside me. I may have not had control over what I was exposed to or what was taught to me growing up, causing such pain and angst, but I do have control now and that is the best way to liberate my life. But before I made the decision to be better than my dad, and better than my mom, I had to face the truth that the very man that had broken me to pieces, who I swore I would never be like, is the very man I was turning into.

Father, NO

For the majority of my life I feared telling you "NO."
The reality was, I needed to tell myself "NO."
My innocence was robbed and the discipline was lost in translation.
A complex back and forth, the sabotage made way.
Falling in love with a lie of who you were, the things you did for me,
just so I   could feel and believe I was loved by you.
A monster you were.
A monster I became.
Father, no.
A light in your heart shattered through the pain.
You chose to be there, and not falter again.
I tell you I love you.
We are always going to be growing and learning from our stain.
We made it this time, so help it to stay.
Father, no. No more fighting for an end.

Chapter 4

#cherrypoppin#whosebirds#whosebees

The gravity of childhood trauma and upbringing can later cause you to act one, if not all, of three ways: fearful, vain, or highly sexual. I am a product of all three. You see, I was one of those children who needed attention and validation SO badly that I made up stories to sound likable, perhaps even cool at times, in hopes that those around me would accept me. It never occurred to me that I could be my authentic self and NOT get ridiculed for it. I forfeited my ability to think on my own and went straight to pathological lying. I had always thought that what I had to say didn't matter and if I had an opinion that was different from anyone else's, I would be branded as dumb or wrong. So I lied. I feared not being able to perform which caused me to 'people please' most of the time. I was more concerned with meeting other people's standards in lieu of my own. In time, I grew vain about having a specific demographic of people to please, ultimately landing me in the overly sexualized category as a result of my fear of failure. I coped with my anxiousness through sex and masturbation. It was my ultimate escape.

I grew up in the '90s and 2000s, and the music and movies out at that time raised me. Movies like *Thirteen* written and directed by

Catherine Hardwicke, and any movie with Angelina Jolie in it, particularly *Gia* by Michael Cristofer, gave me confidence that I hadn't been familiar with. Glamorizing sex and its appeal was something my innocence couldn't quite comprehend, but it seemed like something I could do while out in the real world. Songs like "Right Thurr" by Chingy and Nirvana's "Smells like Teen Spirit" had me overzealous because I wore Teen Spirit deodorant and I walked while swinging my hips. The plethora of influences had me obsessed to the nth degree and I would find myself recreating the cinematic art in my relationships with my friends or alone in my room. I would see my life as if it were a rehearsal for the perfect scene. For me, the climax of my movie was an all-out, drama-filled moment where tears were rolling and relationships shattered. Sex could easily cause that downfall. I had figured that out from experience with my parents' divorce. Sex seemed to always be the offense. It was the money shot.

It's not like a whole lot has changed since that era. The dominion of sex, for me as a young teen, marginalized girls so significantly that virginity was lost in my neighborhood while listening to music about how disposable we were. The subliminal messaging that came with the free form of music around sex, love, and heartbreak had the most profound effect on why I used my emotional responses first. Never mind my rational thinking, the emotions that were elicited by whatever song I was listening to would be how I responded to someone that day and later throughout life. It was my preferred way to communicate with my friends and family, and later, my lovers. Song speaking is what I call it. That's my jam. Literally. Have you ever sent a song to someone because it was easier to express what you were feeling through that song rather than sifting through your own words? The meaning behind the lyrics was what I wanted to convey to my lovers. Whether it be an I hate you, I love you, or I want to sleep with you; music was my voice.

Sex was and still is the hottest, yet most controversial, subject. I believe it is treated like a commodity rather than a privilege. The transaction of sex determined if I was going to feel sacred or unworthy in that moment. I know my parents didn't mention sex as they should have until I was in my thirties with two kids. I believe they missed the mark on that one. They were sexually repressed and it made for a concoction of self-taught children. There was this one time when I was 16 that my mom made me look up every STD on the internet, write a list of them, and study the severity of each disease. I guess she was hoping I would have been educated while simultaneously freaking out over the symptoms, enough to make me think twice. It worked for a little while until I caught my first round of Chlamydia in my 20s, unable to pinpoint who gave it to me and who I gave it to. The phone calls I had to make were excruciating. That was all I got from my mom about sex as she watched me subject myself to bad decision after bad decision.

I had no regrets about the decisions I was making with my sexual encounters, but I did know my heart had been suffering each time I gave a piece of myself away. I knew I was deeply buried in the sorrows of my home life and wanted to feel anything but the pain that came with my family. Once my parents went their separate ways, all I could poke at were the gashes of their emotional abuse. I almost wished they would have beaten me instead. I'd look back and would want constant check-ins over my growth and sexual understanding. Some guidance around self-worth and sex would have been nice, considering how they coincide with one another. I wanted the reason for exploring my sexuality to be of my own accord, not because I was pressured, or worse—forced.

My earliest memory involving sex was being introduced to dry humping by my aunt. Yes, I said aunt. Her name is Shantel. She's a year older than me and is my dad's youngest sister. It was bizarre, I'll admit, knowing my grandma had a child around the same time my mom had me. Shantel would sneak us into my grandma's shed for our sessions together and they would advance each time. The sickness that is sexual abuse wasn't cautioned or known about in my family, even though plenty of us had encountered it, until it was too late. I never spoke a word about going over to my grandma's and playing with Shantel in a sexual manner. I didn't realize that the play we engaged in was inappropriate, even though I had an idea of what we were doing from snippets of information I'd gathered here and there. I wasn't equipped to know much about the multiverse of sexual exploration, but I did know that it felt good and I felt safe since it was with someone I knew. We both were left in a vulnerable position that later manifested in harsh behavior towards each other. It wasn't until I reopened that vault of my childhood experience that I spotted why I wanted more and more sexual attention.

How old were you when you first lost your virginity? It has always been taboo and the world can't seem to get on the same page regarding such an intimate right of passage. Some downplay sex while others put it on a pedestal. Did you know in Mexican culture a father can throw his daughter a party known as a "Quinceanera", quince meaning fifteen, to celebrate a young girl becoming a woman? It symbolizes readiness for marriage in hopes of keeping the tradition alive. I recall really wanting a Quinceanera when I was a little girl. Something about those princess dresses bouncing light off each sequin had me feeling like the only way I could be beautiful or sought after was to be presented at a party with all the bells and whistles. I never got a

Quinceanera and I never bothered to ask why. I guess I really didn't need a party to show I was ready for sex since I had already had sex by the time I was 15, and there was certainly no celebration for it. Never mind teaching me that my developed body was biologically ready for sex, even though my young mind sure as hell wasn't.

The behavior I would display after growing up around the young girls in my family would attract me to partying and attention-grabbing. My family was/is adamant about attending big parties. Shocker, right? Even though my parents didn't really drink, I saw my other relatives indulging in alcohol and food, having a great time getting drunk and dancing. Quinceaneras were always a great time to showcase how adultlike I could be. Getting dolled up was part of the assignment and waiting for someone to compliment me was my A+. I saw the girls in my family wear clothing that showcased lots of skin and jewelry that would bling no matter what angle you stood at. Being so young and wanting big hoop earrings and a bandana over my head to match my crop top and tight jeans seemed normal to me. I remember my dad doing everything he could to protect me from becoming a "Chola", or someone he deemed less than prim and proper. He did his best to keep a close eye on me, but it only made me want more freedom.

As you know, there is such a thing as good AND bad attention, and I didn't care which I got; I wanted both. Whether it was with my style or my attitude, I knew I wanted to be recognized for my efforts. I was an overachiever who got good grades and excelled in my extracurricular activities in hopes that my performance would earn me affection from my parents. They kept me busy and I thought that my ability to perform well would label me worthy in their eyes. Perfection was the priority in our house considering all the time spent looking polished, dressing well, and refining our skill sets. It was hard to depict what was in good moral standing and what was abusive. I should have voiced my concerns sooner with how my constant strides towards accomplishing a single goal, even if it was just my appearance, stressed me out. Even if I had, I'm not sure my parents were capable of listening. Once my parents' marital problems were known, it was harder to get the attention I needed for emotional development and stability. I decided that what I was getting from my peers at school would suffice. I wanted all the friends I could collect. I was a bully after being bullied, and I was a leader just as much as I was a follower. And so it goes - nothing I did would be good enough and my self-worth was compromised.

I remember this one time in the 6th grade when I put an earring through the first few layers of my tongue to make it look like a tongue ring. Classic move, right? I started getting reactions I enjoyed because of how disturbing I was being. I wore lacy panties my mom bought me at Victoria's Secret that would be seen by the boys who sat behind me in class. My dad had enrolled me in a middle school where he was the onsight officer, in hopes of keeping hormone-raging boys away, when in reality it caused a political issue after an outbreak of "M.K. Rave, please come to the principal's office." I eventually got kicked out of that school after the last straw was pulled by causing a fight between two boys. Physical violence over a girl? No way! Each boy claimed I had said yes to being their girlfriend, but in my defense, I had no clue that it wasn't okay to have more than one boyfriend. It was harmless lunchtime handholding, it's not like I was going to marry these boys. My parents were the only model relationship that mattered to me and lying, cheating, and dating multiple people set the tone for a lot of what I later would encounter. I was just practicing what I had learned. After getting kicked out of school, you'd think I'd learned my lesson about causing a scene or cutting back on the boy-crazy tension. Nope. I was only getting started.

I'll never forget the night out at Camy Todd's guest house in the middle of the desert. Her parents were nowhere to be found, which was something I found fascinating. There were a lot of kids from our school and other kids I'd never seen before. I was able to go with my best friend at the time, Jillian Barry. Jillian and I met at Capshaw Middle School before she ended up at a continuation school on account of her truancy. Of course, I would befriend another bad influence to go with my bad influence. This beautiful, blonde-haired, blue-eyed girl only had her mom raising her and that meant she got to do whatever she wanted! Our moms were suffering through the reality of their lives at the same time, so naturally, we bonded over their demise. Jillian and I went to this party where we teens were drinking jungle juice out of a giant bucket. I'll never forget seeing Bomb Pop popsicles floating around in the pool of alcohol. What is it with Bomb Pops??? Those popsicles only heated up the party by being phallic objects to imply a sexual act.

As the night progressed, my supposed sleepover at Jillian's ended with me giving my first blowjob to Camy's boyfriend, Luca, while Camy was passed out next to us in her bed. I had felt a high from being devious that I had never felt before. On top of being drunk for the first time, I felt this euphoric state that would leave me careless about Camy's feelings if she were to find out that her boyfriend cheated on her with me. After that night, I looked for any reason to hang with Jillian when it was my week to stay with my mom. I wanted nothing more than to drink, attract boys, and hopefully get laid for the first time.

I was known as the tease and Jillian was the one that jumped to third base before knowing your last name. She had been more experienced than I, and I was beginning to like the coy manner that attracted people to me. I would kiss you, but not let you touch me under my clothes. I would bat my eyelashes and smile, but not give you my number. I would flash you, but giggle when you walked away with a hard-on. Calling me a prude wasn't true, but I let all the boys think so. You know, the famous line of "I've never done this before," right before I was about to do the repetitive act had me hooked on how easy it was to make people think they were special. After my first BJ[1], I had decided it was too much work to touch boys and I knew I wanted to abstain from going all the way until I found the right guy. It was a ploy to play on their emotions, and I noticed how enthralled I was over it– that and masturbating. Both turned into a ritual for me. No one taught me that I wasn't a mutant for wanting to get creative with how I made myself orgasm, and I vaguely remember a health class in the 5th grade explaining my period and how boys got erections, but nothing about wanting to rub up against everything or how silly boys behaved when you were around them.

It was when I found my dad's vintage Playboy and loved what I saw that I decided I wanted to consciously make an effort toward girls. It was the Marilyn Monroe issue of Playboy and I got sensations that prompted me to touch myself more and more. A woman's body was so attractive to look at– way prettier than the penis I put in my mouth, that's for sure. There was an instance when I crept down the hall and caught my parents watching a porno. In plain view, I saw a woman rubbing ice cubes on her nipples and knew that it stimulated me more than seeing a naked man. It's memories like this that stick with you forever, clearly. I felt I had already had my fun with boys, so maybe it was time to do more with girls. My friends and I would giggle and

---

[1] BJ = blow job

discuss how we wanted to kiss and fondle boys but practiced kissing each other instead when alcohol and peer pressure came into play. I would kiss Jillian at parties because it riled up the boys and the chanting for us to make out was too loud to drown out.

It was a chain reaction. Kissing girls led to kissing guys, and that resulted in clothes coming off. My clothes would come off while on a trampoline one night at Randal Wilson's house. So much for sticking to girls. He was a grade above me and a total skater boy. He had sandy blonde hair and blue eyes with the silliest wardrobe. I thought he was attractive regardless of his oversized white T-shirt and the irony of his beanie worn in the summer. He was the IT SHIT and all the girls wanted him. I liked his cousin, Brian, but he wasn't cool like Randal was. I started to develop a fixation with being "cool" by proxy, even if that meant ditching my true crush on Brian. If I could sit with the cool girls, I would be cool. If I could hook up with the cool guy, I was cool, and a slut, because let's face it, this was middle school. The night before 8th grade graduation I made plans to sleep over at my other best friend's house, Cory Gordon. She and I were celebrating that we were going to be high schoolers and that meant Vodka. Cory was a wild child with a hint of goth and granola. She was a different kind of attractive than me. We had our guy friends over to help us make a dent in the Vodka bottle just so we could later fill it up with water as if her parents wouldn't notice. Alcohol gave me the courage to come out of my shell and say things that I normally wouldn't say, and that alone got me the attention I wanted from Randal.

I loved sounding outrageous and confident when I drank. My elaborate stories gave me a false sense of security and I would cross my fingers and hope that the person I was telling my stories to wouldn't notice I was lying. Lying was my way of ensuring I was cool enough for the friendship, or in this case, to make Randal my boyfriend. Most of my erotic behavior took flight when I drank. Randal was one of the boys that was at Cory's house and Cory noticed Randal flirting with me and became jealous. She kicked all the guys out of her unsupervised living room and made them go home, leaving her and me to drink by ourselves. It was late and she told me that we should go to bed, so we headed for her room where she blasted some Marilyn Manson. Cory suddenly leaned in and kissed me. Soon after her kiss came a push back onto her bed and her sliding my pants to my ankles. I stared up at the ceiling and wondered who Marilyn Manson was because his music was insane, in a good way. I felt hazy and confused. I felt that my submission was in order. The idea of stopping her and not going with the flow made me fear that I would lose a friend. Perhaps this was one example my people-pleasing tendencies to feel accepted.

I became aware, more and more, that there was a specific desire people had to get me in a position for sex, even if I wasn't leading them on, and it felt out of my control. When I would tease and play games with my friend group, I felt in control, but in situations like this one with Cory, I felt helpless. I was caught off guard. After Cory was done going down on me, she came up and whispered "My turn," and my mouth dropped, literally, under the covers. That morning we woke up and acted like nothing happened. We didn't address any part from that night. How casual sex was in the media and now in my personal life kept the justification of random sex alive. "Maybe this is just the way it goes," I would tell myself. I went to my 8th grade graduation the next day and that evening I told my mom I was going over to Jillian's, which we know means I was conspiring with my friends on how to sneak out and go over to Randal's place. I had made up my mind that I was going to have sex with him. No hand job or blow job, but full-on penetration. I had already learned how to use condoms with all the lessons from my friends, so I had that going for me. Knowing Cory took advantage of me at her place jump-started my engine to gain some revenge. How could I not rev towards hooking up with the one guy I knew she didn't want near me– Randal Wilson?

The night sky helped each star illuminate with its deep backdrop as I stared passed Randal's head dangling over me. The pressure was so different from all the other sexual activities I had explored prior to this moment. The bouncing from the trampoline made things seem easier when really I was distracted by it more than I was enjoying it. The disassociation during our sex would later be the protocol for me; I would leave my body on some spiritual level and return once it was over. It was over pretty quickly when Randal rolled to the side of me and began with small talk about the trampoline. We laughed and smoked some pot, which in my opinion was the best part. Randal was sweet when he wasn't around his crew. There wasn't a whole lot of emphasis on sexual orientation or labeling when I was growing up like there is today, but I would eventually end up identifying as bisexual after that night. A month away from turning 14, I had already experienced sex with both a guy and a girl and I knew I was unveiling my capabilities with both; I just wasn't sure which was better or which I liked better. There was only one way to find out and that was to explore more.

The rumors that would percolate before I entered into high school would be some of the heaviest of my young life. I thanked Randal for my vaginal awakening and left middle school with both confidence and timidity. Slut, whore, and "privileged daddy's girl who was going to end up a teen mom" were some of the things said that shaped how I saw myself. Although I did act conceited, like I didn't care about the name-calling, beneath the surface I felt shame for being sexually active, even though I was provocative any chance I got. I couldn't help it. I once walked into a bathroom stall at school and saw "Let's shank M.K." written in black Sharpie marker. I had to ask my friends what 'shank' meant since I was unsure and didn't find it that menacing. It certainly isn't a good thing.

Hearing how I did this or that with some boy ranked me highly unlikeable, even though half of the gossip was untrue. I get it. I know how rumors work and I was guilty of spreading some myself, but when I started to get jumped by girls that looked the way my dad didn't want me to look, I began to understand the power of my words. It was time to prepare myself for the next fight by learning from my father who studied Ju-Jitsu. I wanted my fellow students to know I was tough and ready for anything, and when I wasn't acting like a wannabe, gang-banging chola, I was wearing a pearl necklace and shoelaces to match my polo shirt, secretly waiting for a fight to unfurl. I felt like I was the perfect balance of dangerous and debutant. I noticed the attention I got from boys becasue of it and I ate it up for every meal, every day, and still could not wait to get to school for feeding time. My sex addiction and hunger for violence were starting to form.

Chapter 5

#selftaught#paperorplastic

With all the commotion within my circle of friends that summer before high school started, it was time to explore my options away from them and their body parts. I was getting too comfortable and the lackluster relationships caused some serious boredom. I was in high school now, the ultimate watering hole so to speak. I soon caught the attention of my math teacher's son, Tyler, who was a senior at our school. He would frequently visit the classroom and stand at his mom's desk, acting like he was listening to what she was saying while staring at me, waiting for me to look away. But I didn't. After having sex with Randal, I felt overly confident in taking on an older boy. It was my right of passage to look at ALL the prospects, seniors included. I was at track practice one day, standing on the field, when Tyler called me over. He didn't look like he was dressed for any field activity so I was curious as to what he was doing there. I went over and flirted with him and cracked jokes about how his mom was a horrible math teacher, mentioning his clockwork eye-flirting with me every time he visited her class. After a long gaze with his piercing green eyes, he suggested I ditch practice and go with him for a ride. He was at it again.

His eyes had me hooked. I suspected I had a slight obsession with boys with colored eyes. It was as if I became ensconced with the gleam of color, hypnotizing me into making bad decisions. Have you ever been pulled into a trance by looking into someone's eyes? Someone you knew you wanted to embrace you? It seemed to happened to me every time I saw an attractive male with an eye color that was the opposite of mine. I felt special that he chose me to leave campus and go on a cruise with him. Was it that I was special? Or was it obvious that I was easy to pursue? Either way, Tyler had me weak for him. Not that I had displayed strength when it came to sexually powered interactions, but I couldn't imagine saying "No" to him. I always gave guys way more credit for being dreamy than they really were. As I hopped in his truck, I asked where he was taking me. You could tell that he wasn't sure of what the plan was but he was certain he wanted to go somewhere private. We drove around for 20 minutes until we finally landed at his house. I looked at him and brought up the obvious.

"Isn't your mom here?"

"NO, she'll be home around dinner time, so we have to hurry."

"Hurry?"

He took me back to his room and threw a movie on, so I assumed that's what we would do. Watch a movie on his futon for some laughs and flirting. He leaned in to kiss me and my brain clicked on to glitch mode, which meant there a disconnect between being in the moment and jumping to the future. I wanted the moment to end as fast as it started – that dissociation thing. My eyes were open during the kiss and I remember feeling no pleasure whatsoever, just a slimy tongue. His kiss wasn't awful but I didn't feel any sort of heat from it either. Tyler clearly had been way more into it than I was, but I didn't do or say anything to point that out. I froze. He pulled away and opened his eyes to see me with mine wide open. It didn't phase him at all.

"Do you have a condom?" he asked.

"NO, why would I?"

"I thought we were going to have sex."

Silence.

Tyler frantically looked around his room while I watched in amusement. This signaled he had done this before and a condom was surely under his clothes or in his drawers. Yep, this guy wanted to get laid. He stopped rummaging through his disheveled drawers and gave me the funniest expression. It was a look of panic mixed with horniness. I could tell he was flustered and flushed in the face when he asked if I thought a Ziploc baggie would work. Wow. The desperation was real. A Ziploc baggie? What's next? Is he going to suggest a plastic Target bag or a paper bag from Whole Foods if a Ziploc baggie is nowhere to be found?! I was so shut down and turned off that I couldn't respond with anything other than telling him he should just finger me instead. I felt I owed him something since he went out of his way for me, and I was trying to make up for not having sex. I was too afraid to say no. The suggestion of a baggie had me so thrown that if he was willing to do that, he may go to other extremes to get off.

Fear sank in, but I felt confident that I could shock him with some fighting moves if I had to. For some reason, I couldn't bring myself to speak up or speak my truth but I was capable of kneeing Tyler anywhere my knee would go if I had to. Tyler paused and thought about my offer and decided he didn't want to pass it up. No sooner did his excitement take hold of him than his body came to a halt when he heard the front door of his house open. The horror on his face told me it was his mother. He shuffled his way to his closet door and told me to get in. I walked through a pile of Nike shoes and stood as deep in the closet as I could. His mom had called for him and I heard him open his bedroom door to meet her in the hallway. I couldn't help myself but to giggle. Laughing at serious situations was how I coped with negative emotions. I was genuinely terrified of getting caught. Tyler's bedroom door opened only for me to hear the faint voice of my annoying math teacher. It took everything in me to not pop out of the closet and bust him. He deserved it for his stupid Ziploc suggestion. Fucking moron. Something about having control over getting him in trouble piqued my interest. It sparked something in me to want more power over people who seemed weak in the moment.

I managed to slip out of Tyler's house without being seen and he drove me back to the football field at school just before my mom picked me up. I got out of his truck and snuck back into practice as seamlessly as possible. He drove away with a grin on his face that implied we would try this again. I had to stop and really consider whether or not I wanted to sleep with this bad boy senior, regardless of his stupidity. Something about checking him off my less-than-evolved wish list of things to conquer would make me feel more accomplished. You would think I had some radar for judgment after his bonehead idea, but all inhibition was out the window and my only motive was to push the envelope. I was told by one of my friends that I purposely targeted dumb, sexy guys so I can make them feel inferior to me. I apparently got off on the arousal of pity.

The next day at school I did my best to hunt Tyler down on campus since he failed to reply to any of my texts. Yes, the good ol' days of single-character texting on flip phones. I was already aggravated over how I exerted myself for a drawn-out text message that wasn't met with any response. I was doing my best to engage with Tyler to talk about what happened at his house but he was ignoring me. It was during 2nd period when I was in the library passing notes to my bestie at the time, Kourtney Solis, that something changed. It was normal for Kourtney and I to dish gossip and shit talk through notes formed into hearts or some other origami shape. This particular note wasn't air-dynamic enough to make it to the table where she was sitting since it was swiftly intercepted by our teacher. Luckily it wasn't my math teacher since the note consisted of dirty details that had happened with Tyler. I remember writing "Is it rape when you don't want it to happen?" on the note. The supervising teacher in the library gave me the famous index finger shake back and forth as if I didn't already know I shouldn't be passing notes in class. My stomach fell to the floor and my head rushed with blood as I sat and watched her slowly open the note. Her face turned pale with concern and she did her best to calmly walk over to me to escort me out of my chair towards the door. I looked back at Kourtney and all she could mouth to me was "I'm sorry" for not catching the note.

I walked directly to the school counselor's office where my mom and dad were soon called after the counselor asked me for more details of the story. At this point, I was so afraid of getting in trouble that my instinct was to lie to get myself out of it. I grew up with lying my way out of things and it was the preferred option for me. Once my parents showed up, they had a meeting with my principal and the counselor, without me, and my dad took me to the rape crisis center where he had been many times before since becoming a detective. I was put in a room and examined left and right, when finally a doctor came in to check me out. I thought to myself about how this event with Tyler really blew shit out of water. I was enjoying how attentive people were to my feelings and physical state, but I was so confused as to why everything got overdramatized because a senior touched me and I asked about rape in a note. I didn't state that he DID rape me so why all the fuss?

I minimized the gravity of the situation because of how triggering it was but I didn't know that at the time. No one addressed the real problem of how I got to that place, only how illegal the sexual acts were since it was with an 18-year-old boy. Yes, he was legally an adult but his mind was that of a 13-year-old, that's for sure. Just when you think someone is more mature than you, you find out they aren't. It seemed like the longest day of my life and it would only get longer when an investigator walked through the door and sat down in front of me after his firm introduction of what he was doing there. He had been cross-examining my story since I kept giving different versions of the same thing. I was told that Tyler was going to get in trouble since he was 18 and I was only 14. I was stunned with fear over what was to come of this situation, how embarrassing it would be to go back to school, and most importantly, how angry Tyler was going to be. I didn't want to disappoint him, yet if I had the chance to tell him "That's what you get for not texting me back," I would have.

After all was said and done, I was able to go home and journal about everything. It's not like any of my family members spoke to me about what had happened. There were no check-ins or questions about how

I was feeling over such a controversial situation, and it was as if my parents just shut down. Out of sight, out of mind, and if they did show any care or concern, it wasn't displayed by communicating with me through that traumatic event. What was going to happen to Tyler? I received no explanation, just that he was going to get in legal trouble. I never saw him, or my math teacher at school, again. Whoa. I had no idea the drama that could be caused by doing sexual acts with boys. Ironically, despite having a father who worked with this very subject.

My dad used to work sting operations with me and Kourtney outside of grocery stores to get adult males to buy us alcohol. This was the same father who failed to speak to me about the prowling of males on us young females or about how an 18-year-old boy at school is categorized no different than the 30-something-year-old man who just bought us alcohol on camera. No one sat me down and gave me the "you are a beautiful young lady and you are going to attract a lot of attention from older men who want to touch you and offer you things," talk. I found that out on my own. Not that Tyler is excused from being a dip-shit, but I don't believe what happened between us was rape. I was still unsure of the concept of rape at the time. I had asked the team at the rape crisis center to explain it to me, but it still wasn't registering. Unwanted sexual acts by someone older than me? Legal age? Consent? Statutory rape?! All the terms used to describe such an offense had me bewildered. At this point, I wanted all the sexual acts with the boys of my choosing, and I wanted those acts to be how I envisioned them in my dreams, not how they wanted them. I had successfully controlled the sex I was having with my partners, except with Cory and Shantel, up until this point. I didn't feel taken advantage of nor did I feel the boys I chose were smarter than me. Exploiting weaknesses was how I kept myself safe. I wanted to be in control even though I had no handle on using my voice. I guess that's why it is illegal for older boys to be sexually involved with younger girls—mental and emotional maturity. My inability to say no can attest to my immaturity regardless of how much smarter I thought I was.

My freshman year came to an end and I collected some epic memories of ditching class and going on adventures with my new friends, who were mostly seniors. It all caught up to me when a truancy officer reported me to my principal, who then reported me to my parents. So what? I smoked some weed…ok. Ok…a lot of weed, and went off campus; I wasn't particularly enthused with my classes. I was, however, learning a lot in my social life. I was too busy experiencing plenty of *firsts*! My first time getting dumped by a boy, claiming I was too young for him, was important for my big-headed attitude. He must have heard about the Tyler incident. Or maybe it was because he saw me attempt to smoke my first cigarette in the school parking lot and noticed I had no idea what I was doing. I wasn't completely heartbroken because I was pursued by his friend, Matt, days later. Matt Stratford would go down in history as my first high school love. You know, the kind you write about in your diary with talk of running away together or committing suicide if your parents ever kept you apart. That type of love.

Matt was a senior who had just graduated and I was supposed to be going into my sophomore year. I thought it was appropriate math, him being 18 and me at 14, soon to be 15. I didn't think the age gap was significant, not like Tyler and I with the wapping four years instead of only three. Matt didn't mind either. He always claimed I was "mature for my age." I looked at Matt as if he could provide me with everything I needed, and he was quick to make my world better when I would come to him in tears about my home life or if I just wanted a dopamine hit. He always offered a distraction in some form or another. All the attention I ever wanted, I got from Matt. He would order his friends around to do anything to keep me close to him. "Call and act like her mom and get her out of class!" I was amazed when I asked for something and it was done for me at the snap of my fingers. Having that kind of power only led me to harsh encounters, and hardship after hardship started to arise.

I noticed it was my demands that were getting me into trouble. A constant moan of "I want this, let's do that," was weighing the scale too heavily and it would only get heavier when Matt introduced me to an assortment of different drugs: ecstasy, cocaine, hashish, and mushrooms. I have no idea what the hell Matt was thinking when he let me dabble with such hefty drugs but I came to the conclusion that I didn't like how I couldn't control the outcome when I tried each one. Matt wasn't concerned about being the "good guy" for me, instead taking on the role of the fun guy who just wanted to show me off, get high, and have sex with me was enough for him. Every time I came to him with a problem I wanted to talk through, it was fixed with a party. He knew I enjoyed smoking weed, drinking alcohol, and having sex, so why not offer my addiction as my antidote? Matt and my friend Jill Berry were the most toxic influencers in my life before the term influencer came with a follow button, and they knew I was their biggest fan. Jill had dropped out of school and she and Matt wanted me to follow them into their world of oblivion. I started to, until I met the girl who changed my mind.

I used to tuck myself into bed at night after countless hours of daydreaming about my version of the perfect guy. He would come through my window and wake me up, ever so gently, by kissing my lips and whispering how deeply he loved me. He would tell me how safe I would be if I took his hand and trusted him with everything I am, rescuing me from the rattling of my home life. A certain type of male started to come into existence for me with prominent features. My dream boy from the window. Tall, pale-skinned, green or blue-eyed, with white teeth and a big penis. The six-pack was always a bonus. I would want him to be smart, funny, and driven too, but I was too shallow as a 15-year-old girl to really care if he had those characteristics, I didn't set the bar too high for myself. What a mistake that was. This fantasy of being loved by a romantic guy was alive and active in me, not just because it was what I was taught by the world around me, but because I was longing for security I had never felt before. Being with Matt helped me escape my reality of the brokenness that was created from infancy but it merely perpetuated the pain of my ever-evolving addiction. He was not my perfect guy.

After my truancy officer conspired with my principal in various attempts to challenge me in school to keep me in school, my mom decided that it was time to be homeschooled. Placing me in class with seniors in hopes of stimulating me academically only pushed me to make more friends I could misbehave with. The attitude I gave my mom about being homeschooled was excessive since I was afraid of how I would be judged for being some homeschooled freak. But the moment she told me I would be home by myself during the day, I changed my tune. At this point, I was a sophomore in a homeschooling program living with my mom full time. My dad and I had one of our many falling outs, so he wasn't a part of my life to say otherwise. My mom was an "easy, breezy, beautiful cover girl" and allowed me to have more freedom than I should have. Can you blame her? I'd be scared of me too. I took on the role of the house terrorist. I got what I wanted when I wanted it, and if not, pandemonium would ensue and my mom would be in tears. My stepfather knew not to come anywhere near the drama since he had failed to raise his own three daughters who weren't a part of his life at the time. Until a phone call changed everything.

I was content with my life as a homeschooled student with the internet as my teacher, sleeping most of the day, except the days I threw pancake parties for my friends in hopes they would ditch class to come see me, and having the freedom to work at my own pace. Life seemed to be on my terms and it made me feel like an adult. I did most of my school work late at night and smoked weed and played pretend during the day. It was like I was six all over again with my imagination running wild. I had way too much time to create fable stories to share with the world. MySpace had been out at the time, and what better way to showcase my stories than with strangers on the internet? I used to form fake relationships with other teenage boys. I called them fake because I would overexaggerate my feelings for them just to gain a reaction. It seemed easy to do when hiding behind a screen. That sort of thing is more than relevant today but I hadn't realized that I was, in fact, catfishing by exploiting vulnerability in others for my own amusement.

I would dare myself to venture out and test the waters of my ambiguous behavior with all the freedom of being home alone; I would tamper with the dangers of the internet. My insensible behavior would suggest that what I was doing was harmless when in actuality, I was harming people alongside myself. The evil I began to dally with was more than just a subtle nuance. I would make decisions to mess with people based on how I was feeling. If I was angry, I would lash out and attempt to bring someone down by affecting their mood with my words. If I was happy, I would fish for compliments and shop for a cute boy to potentially hook up with. The people I interacted with were nothing more than subject matter to me, and I used them to make my escape from reality worthwhile. All I really wanted, more than a reaction to people's demises, was to lustfully play in my jungle gym of wonderment. I was too young to stamp myself as a sadist, but I did love taunting boys with my feminine features and mishandling their emotions. It came easy when I flaunted the fact that I was a model.

It was when I started modeling that I began to exhibit my femininity as if my importance was based on my beauty. I had been modeling for a few years and had been actively dancing since I was a young girl. I loved entertaining people by being on stage and it began when I studied ballet at a local dance studio. I practiced other dance forms before enrolling in a belly dancing class at a college for an extracurricular activity. I knew I wasn't going to make an exceptional ballerina since my hips and thighs grew double in size. Belly dancing seemed to be a perfect fit for me, igniting my passion for sex with sheer sensuality; it seemed this genre of dance was made for me and all the mischief I had planned to use on guys. I was reluctant at first to show anyone what I had learned in class until I took a hit of herb and mustered up the courage to show my friends how sexy I could be. During my performances at parties or recitals, I noticed the sensations I got throughout my body and I loved it. From my head to my toes, I knew I felt a rush from dancing and it began to feel like a vice.

Dance Thrills

I have the light creeping in through the window
as it hits my body to highlight my favorite accents.
My torso rolls with separated muscles and all I think at that moment
is…
that I wish he could see me.
The real me.
I dance alone in my space to my music with every beat flattering my
flesh in the
most delicate way.
I want his eyes to follow my enticing curves.
They speak.
A gentle but inviting *hello.*
I gaze upon my hands as they tell a story to draw him near me.
I inhale a wish,
swallow a dream,
and exhale a desire.
Pushing my breath toward him as if he were here, in front of me.
He blinks, and I speed up.
Catch your breath and feel the heat wave hit.
Moving fast is something I've always done,
but it is this type of movement that is the only way it has proven
to work.

The duality of being confident in front of the masses and insecure
with people one-on-one would be apparent to me as I continued my
walk of exuding sexual prowess. I look back on my inability to get close
to anyone on an emotional level and question why I had no trouble

being intimate with people on the level of seduction. I could arouse you and show you my naked body, but I couldn't share my secrets with you or the very depths of my heart. See, I learned that if you just behaved like the world owes you something, people gave you things like they owed you, thus deflecting from having to open up. Modeling and dancing were the perfect scapegoats for my angst and heartache. Masking the complexities of my tangled feelings came easily with modeling and dancing as my outlet. I would express myself through the camera as if I were taking back control of the life that was robbed from me, and I would dance through the shame I felt of being identified as a nymphomaniac by my friends and boyfriends.

Traditionally, men were supposed to sleep with more women than women sleeping with men, but in my case, I had given all the males around me a run for their money. I refused to see how my drive for sexual tension caused damage I wasn't ready for. Are we ever ready to be severely hurt by the damage we cause? The push and pull I had with the people closest to me was how I thought relationships were supposed to be. I would reel you in and whisper sweet nothings in your ear just to throw you out like yesterday's trash. The dynamic of my love affairs and how I responded to my true feelings would change when she moved in.

Chapter 6

#badsister#sussaf

When someone would ask me what I wanted to be when I grew up, I would always tell them something different. It was a wide range of things! I wanted to be a model, rockstar, choreographer, and writer. I wanted to direct movies, act in movies, be on stage, and also be a journalist for some big-time magazine. I had such big dreams that I wasn't about to let anyone confine me to a box. I hadn't realized that I was the one putting myself in a box by limiting myself to addiction. I didn't know I was an addict though. How could I? I was 16 and living my best life, regardless of all the drama unfolding around me. Exhibit A: My newly found stepsister.

My mom and stepdad, Andy, received a phone call from his ex with whom he had a daughter, and all of a sudden, this 13-year-old girl dropped in my lap like some stray cat. I could not fathom having a stepsister, especially knowing she would have to bunk with me! How dare they! It was the ultimate breach of privacy and without missing a beat, I threw a fit. After moving a twin bed into my room, it was time to invite the charity case over.

"Be nice, M.K., and treat her with manners. Make her feel like she's right at home," my mom said to me in her famous patronizing fashion. I was more than ready to make her life so unruly that she would want to go back to her podunk town in Oklahoma.

It had been a regular, homeschooled day for me when my parents showed up at the house with my brothers and a thin, dark-skinned girl with a prominent beauty mark on her chin. Her name was Zieya. I was in my room on my bed with my laptop open and all the appropriate accouterment of a teenage brat. I heard a knock on my door as it was opening; as if I had any other choice than to say "Come in." It was my mom and Zieya standing in the doorway. I met eyes with my new roommate. She was short with dark, curly hair and a look that insinuated she was both pissed off and scared. I shut my laptop aggressively as if I had something to hide and said "Hey" in the most annoying pitch I could think of. My mom suggested we get to know each other and left the room in a hurry so she could go wrangle my brothers before dinner. Zieya sat on her bed and in the first few sentences she spoke, she would have me utterly speechless.

"Wow, you're really hot."

"Uh…thanks. You're pretty too."

"I like your room."

"I like it too. Your outfit's cute."

"I'm not some little girl you are going to have to watch out for. I can take care of myself."

"Ok, I've never had a sister-type person around so....this is new for me."

"Let's just be friends then."

"I like that, let's be friends."

After an evening of skipping the dinner table and settling into our new setup, Zieya and I spent hours talking and briefing each other about our lives. It was 3 AM when we finally shut off the valve and fell asleep. I was used to being nocturnal, but she had to go to my old middle school that morning and I didn't want her to hate her first day, so naturally I took over as her fashion assistant and let her borrow my clothes. As strange as it was, I felt excited to have another girl to share my stuff with. I was always passive-aggressive with other girls, so when I was genuine and honest with Zieya, my anxiety began to dissipate. I hated girls, for the most part, and the majority of them hated me, but Zieya didn't. She was able to hold a conversation of substance and had a cumbersome upbringing that forced her to mature quickly. She didn't hesitate to open up and tell me how it came to be that she was living with us now, and how she had already smoked weed and drank alcohol and had sex. Other than the despairing reality of those facts, I was glad she was on the same level as me. Or at least somewhere close.

Each day after Zieya would come home from school, we would catch up on our current events and gossip. She would fill me in on her world and I felt safe to let her in on mine. That included the nights that I would sneak out and go raving. She knew she had to stay behind but never outed me to my mom. I could tell she had a serious case of FOMO (fear of missing out) but I always assured her that once she was a little older, I would take her with me. Zieya always opted in for hearing about my scandalous nights of rolling on E[1] and having sex, but I never thought the impact of my storytelling would be a reason for her to fight for my attention. There was this time I crept back in through my window after a night of debauchery when Zieya crawled into my bed and began to cry. I lay next to her with both of our heads on my pillow and rolled in to hug her, covering her in a trail of glitter and neon paint.

"Are you ok? Why are you crying?"

"I missed you."

"Awe, I'm right here."

"I don't like that you go out and party without me and hook up with guys."

"I told you we can party together one day. We can smoke some weed right now if you want to?"

"No. I mean, I think that you are too beautiful to be letting guys have sex with you and I hate that they don't know how to love you like I do."

"What do you mean? Are you saying you don't want me to have sex?"

___

[1] Stands for taking/being high on Ecstasy

"Not with them!"

I grew more confused by the second with our conversation as I lay there coming down from the drugs and alcohol. I felt like I was melting in my bed with each blink as I stared at Zieya staring at me. That's when the unthinkable happened. Zi nuzzled my nose and puckered her lips up toward mine. I didn't do anything to stop her.

I woke up later that day, and she was gone to school. I only had a slight haze of what happened at the rave but a clear recollection of the kiss I shared with Zi. Did that really happen? Did Zieya and I make out? Passing out with no memory after we kissed would lead to some questions when she got home. No sooner than I had that thought, Zieya was bursting into the bathroom flailing her arms at me for a hug! I was still in my towel and the steam was thick enough to choke you. I kept my composure as if our kiss was just a figment of imagination. Zieya gave me a big smile and told me how much she enjoyed last night. My face rushed with blood and I did my best to change the subject. I told her to pass me the lotion and I started to lotion my legs. It did not phase her one bit that I was doing everything to avoid the conversation; she kept rambling on about how we should just hook up with each other as if it was some casual thing. Never mind that she's my stepsister - she went on and on about us being an item.

I told Zieya that we could be free-range stepsisters. We both laughed at whatever I meant by that and she reiterated, asking me "Can we hook up, make out, and be each other's dirty little secret?" I knew it would only be possible if we kept it as hush as possible. Our parents could NOT find out, no matter what. I genuinely found Zieya to be attractive; she was so soft and gentle that I appreciated how she treated me as if I were soft and gentle too. I knew I should have put up a fight and said "NO" yet again, but I had been the first girl Zieya ever hooked up with, and it was hard to ignore how in love she was after our first kiss. After all, we were just two teens who want love and sex. Again, I saw nothing wrong within the confines of our own little world, but obviously, this type of relationship is unorthodox and frowned upon – for good reason.

I had agreed to lay off sneaking out and doing drugs after a pep talk from Zieya about how I needed to respect myself and realize that not every guy should get a piece of me. That they weren't worthy. Can you believe this came from a 13-year-old? I was so taken aback by how she fueled my self-esteem that I had quit raving and sleeping with guys, for the most part, with the exception of the virginity I felt obligated to take from a neighborhood boy up the street. Zieya seemed to have hated guys with all her might and there wasn't any level of the male species that could keep her away from me. It could have been Paul Walker jumping off my poster and landing in her bed, and she wouldn't give him a second look. I was it for her. That's all it took before it came crashing down.

My mom and Andy had a strange marriage from the moment they met; I knew something was off. After my mom won the custody battle over my brothers, she decided to move back to her hometown, my hometown, in Yellow, Texas. Andy wanted to stay in New Mexico since it was his stomping grounds, and now that his daughter was back in his life, he had no plans to up and leave. Mom moved me to Yellow first before transitioning everyone else. Andy agreed to stay behind and sort things out with his job which meant Zieya and I would be separated. I had learned to numb myself with the assurance that I would find another cuddle bug or fuck buddy as soon as I got to where I was going. In my mind, I could replace Zieya with hopes I wouldn't face the fallout of my real feelings being shredded to pieces. Needless to say, I was apathetic towards the whole situation. I told Zieya goodbye and not to worry, she'd see me again soon.

I was 17 now and living wild and free in TX with my crazy boyfriend Christian. Yes, the ex-husband that went A-WOL. I had been living with my grandpa Ernest, who was the best thing that could have existed for my brothers and me, a real, male figure we could look up to with his down-to-earth personality. Nothing would do justice to how loud his heart was and the way he loved was as if he couldn't help it. I was done with school and my mom and I were constantly butting heads since Grandpa Ernest would let me get away with murder while she did her best to keep me reeled in. It was over a fight that she blurted out how concerned she was for me after Zieya had ended up in the hospital under a suicide watch. I hadn't known. I felt like I was doing a decent job by checking in on her and letting her know I loved her, so I was beyond shocked when I found out. That wasn't all my mom had spilled.

Evidently, Zieya was checked into a facility and was keeping a journal, as we angsty girls do, and in that journal was every detail of her and I coming together romantically. A nurse found the journal, read it with blatant disregard for Zieya, and reported it to her dad. Andy called my mom, and my mom told me. I stared at my mom when she asked me if it was true. We locked eyes, and to prevent tears from trickling down my face, I shook my head with disgust and said "Ew, no!" and walked away. I cried myself to sleep that night and all hell broke loose after that moment. It was as if the only person who really cared for me, who really loved me, I let down by leaving her behind. I felt like I needed to rescue her, but after that bombshell my mom dropped, I knew things would never be the same again.

A couple of years went by and Andy had finally been living with my mom in TX, without Zieya, after the allegations of us sleeping together. It's no wonder they didn't want us to ever see each other again. He left Zieya in New Mexico with his mother after she had been released from the medical center. Andy had already abandoned her once when she was little, so what did it matter if he was leaving her behind again? I knew the feeling. Zieya had been released but was under her grandma's watch. However, somewhere in my skewed judgment, I thought it would be a great idea to kidnap her. How bad could it be since she was almost legal? Zi was able to contact me from her cousin's cell phone, and the plan came to fruition when I traveled 45 minutes away to intercept her as she made a run for it from a window at her grandmother's house.

It was time to exhaust all efforts to make her disappear by inventing a new identity for her. The long black locks she had were chopped off at the shoulder and dyed blonde. Fake glasses and a new name would do the trick. All my friends chimed in to help me hide her so we could be together. I had been actively dating a woman named Alana, as well as making my second round of love efforts with the guy I lost my v-card to, Randal, alongside some other guys I forgot to conquer when I was younger. There was something about revisiting men whom I didn't have sex with when I was a tween and wanting them later as an adult. Have you ever been sweeping and you realize you missed a spot so you go back and sweep up the spots you missed? I wanted to comb through lost desires and gauge whether or not I was still desirable by these people. I was ego-tripping like never before when Zieya would come to save me from myself, and I dropped everyone I was involved with as if I had never met them. She was the only one that meant something to me.

It would seem that Zieya was going stir-crazy and our parents had no suspicions that she was with me, so I felt comfortable in letting her go out with a group of my closest guy friends while I was preparing to leave town. For the record, I've never been able to have a guy friend in my life who honored all the friendship codes and didn't try/want to sleep with me or Zieya. I should have known better than to think otherwise. I had a photoshoot scheduled in Dallas and I gave Zi some instructions before I leff since she wasn't coming with me. What was most important was to keep off the radar and not get caught, or our time together would end once more. I left for Dallas and I got a phone call from the State Police about Zieya being spotted with me and how I should turn her over to them as soon as possible. I, without missing a step, let them know I had no idea what was going on and assured them she wasn't with me. I rushed to get off the phone and immediately called Zi when my friend Warren picked up. I'm told he and Zi decided to take a quick trip to CA for a weed run. She wanted him to leave her there. Unknownst to me, Warren and Zi had been sleeping with each other, so that made him obligated to give her what she wanted, and that was to stay behind in CA.

I get a phone call from the State Police again, demanding that I come into the station for an interview, and so I complied and assured them that I would go to the station as soon as I got back into town. There I was, sitting at a table, being interviewed by the very men who saw me grow up. "Where is she, M.K.?" You bet your ass I lied through my teeth. I had no idea of her whereabouts and I only knew that she was with some guy named Warren Maez. Hell yeah, I'm throwing one of my closest guy friends under the bus for taking Zi across state lines and hooking up with her. I wasn't in a position to be the good guy, but I sure wasn't going to be the bad guy - aside from all the manipulating and lying of course. It would seem as if I had to stay out of her life for good this time. The risk of getting in trouble with the law, or worse, having my heart broken by someone who made me feel like I was someone, is what kept me away. I left the station shaking my head and told myself, "Leave her alone, for good, this time."

Emily Dickinson once wrote a poem titled *I'm Nobody! Who are you?* That plays with the expression of the freedom of anonymity and how we forcefully feel the need to be "somebody" in public and for others. I believe Emily's words were for advocating joy and bliss found within ourselves, not through someone recognizing us and labeling us as "somebody." I didn't know at the time that my happiness wasn't attained through another person. I desperately wanted to mean something to someone, and Zieya held me on a pedestal as if I meant the most to her. Even though she left, I knew she loved me, and it was time to find someone else who would obsess over me the way she did. I'm glad she went off to find her own journey outside of my substance abuse and sex addiction.

I always used my emotional instability as my patsy. The side of me that got drunk and high was the product of my split personality. I only operated on a spectrum of two extremes…really rational or really irrational. I didn't believe there was an in-between. I knew I was indecisive and I began to long for balance. Was I willing to learn about moderation and why it was just out of reach? No. Putting in the work wasn't a priority for me. There's this proverb from the NA (Narcotics Anonymous) handbook that expresses how "one is too many, and a thousand is never enough," and that has proven true in my life. I could never just have one drink; I was always drinking until I blacked out. I could never have one lover, it had to be as many as I could get away with. My addiction was the axiom for why I never finished anything I started, relationships included, and why I was constantly on the move.

There was this one time, I squeezed my eyes shut while my index finger moved around in a circular motion on top of a map of the U.S. I stopped somewhere on a crinkle, only to open my eyes to see where I would be moving next; what I would surround myself with next. There was this antsy feeling I would get that pushed me to run, both literally and metaphorically. I was always being judged by the very people who preached about how I shouldn't harshly judge others, about staying put and doing something with my life. It was a paradox to me. I couldn't seem to make everyone happy so I just did my own thing, which was run. Why do people have a tendency to do the opposite of what they believe? Discern just enough to attract people who are good for you, but don't judge too much, or you're a fascist piece of shit. I just decided to hang with everybody: elitists, bums, child molesters, and famous musicians. I was in no position for boundaries, much less healthy ones. Let's not forget everyone in-between. This sort of attraction I calculated was to prove how I could fit in anywhere. No one had ever rejected me at that point in my life, and I felt more accepted in the outside world using my looks than I did at home with my title as a daughter.

I was living my life on only two volumes: really high or really low. I never grasped the concept of attracting what you are at the time, so I would blame other people for why the temptation was there for me to falter. It's not like I didn't want a break from the burning flavor of Captain Morgan down my throat or a moment of silence from lashing out at my sexual partners for their, and my own, incompetence. It seemed like there was no reprieve from it all. So instead of fighting my addiction, I leaned into it. With Zieya out of my life I was going to drown my reality out after all the people I had cycled through to that point.

It's sad to think how I carried around the people I was involved with like a charm bracelet I wore around my wrist. My accessory to fidget with when I couldn't sit still with myself. I felt I needed to recover from my wild living, but I wasn't ready to learn how to stop. I look back at some of my decisions as a cry for help. I was doing my best to survive by using people for whatever they would give me. Exhausting people for their resources was wearing thin and it was a matter of time before I would drain them, get knocked off my high horse with rejection, and find an alternative way to survive aside from just smiling and pleading. It was my pride that kept me going but begging that kept me using.

So there I was, at my dad's house right before Christmas, when he refused to look at me as anything other than a drug addict who was going to steal his prescriptions from his side of the "his and hers" mirror cabinet. I was done living on couches and raving every night and wanted a place of my own. After that visit, all I could think to do was to rally some money and find a place to rent on Craigslist. Who would help me move since my dad was too busy cheating on his second wife and scorning me? It was time to call Leo.

Chapter 7

#Meet#Cheat#Repeat

It was Christmas Eve and I was dressed to impress with a promising feeling that I'd be swept off my feet, not just because I was going to get laid, but because I was going to portray the perfect *damsel in need of her savior* at the party. I was prepared to set off signals that hyped up my attempts to be noticed, no different than double tapping for that red heart to induce my self-worth. I wanted all the "like" buttons. Jillian was throwing her annual Christmas Eve party at her downtown home, and there was word that Leo was going to be there. My stomach was fluttering with butterflies at the thought of seeing him outside of my sweatpants and messy bun. Leo had helped me move out of Carla's house into my new place, so him seeing me in my red, silk, baby-doll-style dress was going to draw him near as my fairytale, window man.

Leo walked into the party with his friend J.T. and I immediately muttered "Shit!" under my breath. J.T. and I had a threesome with Skarlette one night after watching one of the most fucked up movies I'd ever seen, *Requiem for a Dream* directed by Darren Aronofsky. Nothing like a twisted psychological thriller to get you in the mood. I ignored J.T. just enough to keep him at bay while watching Leo watch me. Leo circled me all night like a hawk, ready to plummet toward his prey. He did to me what I usually do to others. But I was ready for him if he decided to swoop in for the kill. I made sure I didn't drink too much to keep it classy enough to have sex worth remembering, nothing wild, but something he would crave again. Over time, I developed this costume of sexual presence that I thought people would desire and did my best to emulate that. If it was a kink that needed to be explored, I was there for it. If it was the first time for a new act that they weren't sure about, I was there to hold their hand and jump in head first. It turned me on to push the limits with my sex partners. Leo was not someone to be pushed.

I ended up at Leo's house with my high heels kicked off next to his bed and wearing a pair of his socks and underwear. He let me borrow a shirt too since I wasn't prepared with PJs for our sleepover. I sat on his kitchen counter while he made us grilled cheeses to soak up the rainbow of alcohol sitting in our stomachs. He poured us some champagne to wash down our sandwiches as I stared him down and shivered over his suave attitude. He had me ready to crawl under his covers to hold him tight. I didn't care if he had just been texting Carla "I love you" or who he slept with the night before; my eyes were set on this boy and I knew once we had sex, he'd be mine. He took me to his bedroom and we snuggled like two bugs in a rug. I remember him being patient and letting me make the first move to initiate sex. I would have if I hadn't fallen asleep on his chest.

I underestimated how full and drunk I was considering I couldn't stay awake long enough to take our make-out session to second base. It was when I woke myself up snoring that I rushed in to make a move to avoid embarrassment. I seemed to always evade embarrassment by distracting whoever I was around with something sexy. Flipping my hair, a smirk while biting my lip, or my famous side eye with each expression melting my opponent, so whatever silliness sprung my embarrassment would flee. I found myself nestling in his neck for a kiss, and I wasn't going to pass up my chance to let Leo experience what I had to offer. The sun broke through the window in his room as my body met his. An exchange of words would leave us sorry for ever opening our mouths.

I had an opportunity to rent a house out in the middle of the Pecos Mountains when a friend and his family heard about my situation and offered their property out of pity. I guaranteed them I would keep everything kosher since I wasn't going hard with alcohol-poisoned nights or snorting lines of cocaine in the shape of my initials. I lied. It was just days later that Leo had his car filled with his stuff ready to move into my place so we could party together whenever we wanted. So much for having my own space for some much-needed introspection. I understood the power of the pussy, but damn, he fell hard and quick. After the last box was unpacked, Leo wasted no time dropping the L-word over a beautiful ballad with his acoustic guitar. I was smitten over such an extravagant gesture, but I hardly knew the guy. I couldn't help but be more infatuated with the image of him on top of me rather than the invasive statement of "I love you." I had been privy to the term, even when I didn't particularly mean it or understand the merit of saying I love you; it was something I flung around like beads at a Mardi Gras party rather than a deep, mutual exchange with evidence to back it up. All I had to show when it came to my love was the way I gave Leo my body.

Slow-motion sex while kissing passionately or saying his name while moaning a fake orgasm didn't mean I was going to stay loyal to him. It also didn't mean I wasn't willing to try. I wanted him to know my struggle with being fully present in our "love" game we had going on, but how could I possibly share that with him? If I did, it meant he would have all the power for his next move in the game. I say game because that's what I viewed it as. Just like I was a pawn for my parents, I was now a knight moving two steps ahead and one step to the right to avoid letting myself love anyone, especially Leo. I placed myself strategically on the board so I could slip through the cracks and avoid making any real connections. I didn't want to give love in the form of exposing my queen. I'd rather take – take, take, take – and if I ever gave anything back to the relationship, it wasn't in the form of mutual respect. Sure, I was creative with my sexual exploits and met Leo's every need in that category, but I wasn't interested when he tried to open up with me about who he was as "Leo".

I preoccupied Leo with a housewarming party, which he was pumped about since he wanted to showcase us as a couple. I loved that he was always willing to put up with my antics and let me keep the party going every weekend for months straight. I couldn't help myself; I loved the ambiance of a good party. Laughing, crying, making new friends, beer pong, and eating trash food was the regimen of my nightlife and I loved it. But that also meant that a mess was to follow and Leo would be the first in line to help clean it up. There was one mess that he wouldn't dare touch, a mess that would keep us toxic with each other for the next eight years–Zieya.

I had taken an apprenticeship position at a tattoo shop (a fitting environment since I had been getting tattooed at a steady pace since I was 18) and got a new piercing every time I had a mental breakdown. I had a handful of friends who were aspiring tattoo artists who would make house calls to practice their work on me– I was in no position to turn down free ink. I was addicted the moment the needle scraped my skin. Leo happened to be one of those tattooing friends. Most of the artwork on the left side of my body I referred to as my personal coloring book since it was all practice work made up of scribbles and colored outside the lines. I have a range of rudimentary line work to pristine pieces done by well-known artists. It was during a courtesy tattoo from my boss at the studio, who pampered me with free ink in hopes I would sleep with him, that a group of guys strutted into the shop. It was in my job description to be the face of the shop, so I hopped off the tattoo table, pranced to the front desk, and greeted two predominantly white guys and one dark-skinned boy with the most beautiful contrast of green eyes and dark hair. What a smile! I felt like I was ready to have his babies right then and there. This man was that genetically blessed.

It's absurd to think that looks are random. I believe it's a total accident, to some degree, that being "attractive" by earthly standards isn't planned; we have no say in it. I'm given the face I'm given and that's that. I would soon know that this guy named Ara didn't get his looks from his parents because I made him my boyfriend for the next four years. After saying hello and introducing myself, I exchanged numbers with Ara and began an affair with this exotic-looking human. I knew that up to that point, I hadn't had a healthy romantic relationship, but I wasn't going to stop my movie romance from happening by falling head over heels at first sight. Lust is a hell of a drug.

Leo was insanely attractive with his bravado and talents. He was buff and covered in tattoos with a lip ring. I couldn't help but tongue it when I kissed him. Leo did, however, have brown eyes, and I couldn't connect with him as I did when I stared at Ara. I had heard that eyes were windows to the soul and Leo's were dark and cloudy. I learned that Ara was Mexican-American just like I was, naturally making us have a lot in common. I felt like my dad would accept him since he and his family were from the same neck of the woods in Mexico as mine were. I, for once, was elated about impressing my dad with a boy, even though my dad and I were always on the outs with each other. Marrying a white guy didn't help. I had never dated my own kind before since I was usually attracted to men with colored eyes and pale skin who all seemed to have sexual trauma with other men at some point in their past. I wasn't aware back then that it was a damaging factor for all these men I would date, ultimately leading to abusive behavior. I had something in common with Leo, Ara, and all the other men I had been with– sexual trauma.

I wanted to invite Ara to one of my parties so I could show him how important I seemed to be and impress him with how sought-after I was. Keeping Leo and Ara away from each other would be impossible, so I schemed to keep Leo from coming home until Ara left. I told Leo that my dad and I were trying to work through our differences and I was going to have him over for dinner. Leo was aware of the circumstances with my dad, plus he knew who my dad was outside of being just my dad, the big man on campus and with Leo's bad boy rap sheet, he couldn't disagree with my plan. I would have done anything to make this work. I invited Ara and his two friends over after sunset. I had until midnight to seal the deal with him. My version of a deranged Cinderella. No pumpkins, just puppets.

Ara and I had some drinks together and flirted until the tension was just too much to bear. Tons of people were well aware I was with Leo, so I had to dodge them with Ara by my side. We slithered our way to my room where we stood in front of my mirrored closet, looking at the bed through the mirror that was behind us. We shared the same thought. Our first kiss was powerful. His lips were as big as mine and I felt the bounce back at first. All it took was a slight tug on his belt to let him know I was all in, and we fell back on the bed with our reflections giving us a live-action view of what we were about to do next. I should have thought about Leo. How this was our bed and how much he seemed to want this relationship, but I didn't. The only thing I wanted was to experience what I thought was the most handsome man I'd ever seen.

It wasn't long before it was over. No condom, no orgasm for me, just an audition sample of what Ara was in for if he and I agreed to be lovers. Ara buckled his belt back up and walked out of the room first. I was surprised he didn't notice the amount of evidence that suggested a guy also lived in that room, but I guess the pair of men's shoes by the closet didn't keep him from leaning in to kiss me. I know I had plenty of chances to stop, but I didn't, and I will forever be fascinated with the grip sexual cravings have on people—on me. It would keep me in a headlock for years to come. Ara left just in time before Leo got home to wonder why there was a party going on. I told him it was to celebrate that my dad and I fixed things and I was in a good mood. Leo bought my lie, almost every lie. He believed that I met a new friend named Stacy, and every time a text would light up my phone, he thought I was talking to a girl as opposed to a guy I had been sleeping with whom I disguised as Stacy (short for ecstasy). I felt nothing short of ecstasy when I was with Ara.

Leo was my grounded boyfriend who worked hard, was meek at times, and was insistent that touches of romance were a love language. Ara was my rugged mountain man with a taste for adventure that tirelessly pushed me to the ledge, literally. There I was again, in a love triangle, but this time, it was a secret. Unlike Trevor and Skarlette, these two men had no idea I was dating them both. I had never juggled two men before for longer than a day, and I was ready to milk it for as long as I could. I fell in love with how it felt to be looked at and loved differently by Leo and Ara. It was a surprise to me how well I was able to hide them and keep them separate - until I mixed them up. Something of a Freudian Slip. It was only a matter of time before I would refer to Leo as Ara or Ara as Leo. I was walking on thin ice before the unthinkable would happen to trip us all up.

I got a phone call one evening while on the bed with Leo, our legs wrapped together like a pretzel. I released my grip and sat up with a stunned wave of discomfort. It was Zieya. She had still been in California and wanted to come see me. Leo was up to date with my Zieya scenario and had every reason to not want to overcomplicate our relationship by involving her. All it took was one flick of my eyelashes and a hint at a threesome if he would just agree to put her on a Greyhound to come visit me. It took less than 48 hours for Zieya to be boarded on a bus and shipped to me like some Amazon package. Add to cart and confirm payment. I wasn't surprised how easy it was to get what I wanted, and that was the dangerous part of it all. Giving a single person so much power has never been credited to be healthy, and in my case, all the credit for orchestrating such havoc would be paid in the ultimate consequence.

I made sure to organize a welcome home party for Zi; would you expect anything less? Once Leo and I picked her up from the bus station, I knew right away Leo was as captivated by her as I was. I hugged her and kissed her on the lips, with my eyes closed, and then introduced her to Leo. They hugged as if they couldn't wait to do that naked. I felt like bringing us all together would place a flame back in my heart to love again, the self-love I had always forgotten. We drove back to our deserted house in the mountains and caught each other up with what had happened since I last saw her. We both expressed some heated emotions around Warren but decided to put it aside so we could have fun and party for the night. It was over mixed drinks and a couple of cigarettes that I told Zi that Leo and I were up to moving her in with us and becoming a thruple. Zi glared at me with the same look she gave me years ago when I would tell her about my lovers and she'd reply with a "No."

She didn't want to stay but she expressed that her intention for the trip was to get me to go back with her to CA. I had a boyfriend, a secret lover, and now Zi. I was in no position to leave but I told her I would think about it. For now, I suggested we go inside and tag team Leo. We went back inside and I ended up in my bedroom with Zi and Leo putting me to bed. The last thing I saw before fading into oblivion was both their faces hovering over me before I sealed my eyes shut until morning. My alcoholism has always been a crutch for facing the truth. I didn't want to let anyone know what my hopes were: to have my cake and eat it too. Keep Ara, live with Leo, and have Zi all to myself.

The next morning I was greeted with kisses by Leo and Zieya telling me to meet her in the shower. I felt like I was a teenager all over again, hiding the truth about why Zieya and I always showered together. I apologized to Leo first about blacking out and he didn't seem to be disappointed one bit. "Had he and Zieya hooked up without me?" I thought. I met Zi in the bathroom and that is when she told me she didn't want me to be with Leo. She walked me through her thought process on why she thought he wasn't right for me and that he was a douche. I was baffled and didn't know how to respond, so I totally forgot to ask her if they hooked up. It would seem that that wasn't a thing since she was so anti-Leo. What happened last night that would make Zi feel so strongly about Leo in a negative light? I was too hungover to try to sort through everything so I left it alone. Zieya was only in town for a couple more days and I wanted to spend those days showing her a good time. I first had to check in with Ara and tell him that I was going out of town for a bit, but I'd see him when I got back. My life was exhausting.

My drastic lifestyle choices would lead to dramatic scenes like this one…on Zieya's last night, she got so drunk she ended up in the hospital with alcohol poisoning, but not before first spilling her guts about how she didn't like Leo and how she wanted me to run away with her to CA. She pleaded with me to dump Leo and go with her in front of Leo. I was mortified. I looked at Leo as my safe space. He took care of me and my needs, and if I left with Zi, that would all go away. I reassured Leo I wasn't going to leave him and that left Zi in a drunken stupor, facing the reality of me not choosing her over him. It was about 4 AM when she was rushed to the E.R. by my friends since I couldn't take her myself. If we were seen together, we both would be busted for what had happened when I kidnapped her. She was months away from being 18, but I couldn't risk it. I felt like a piece of shit watching her leave in the back seat of some car with the condition she was in.

I kept checking in on her through my friends to make sure she was recovering, and when she was released, they took her to the bus station. Just like that, she was out of my life again. Had I made a mistake? Should I have gone with her? I knew I loved her but I was too shallow to pass up on Leo taking care of me versus me taking care of her. I didn't know how to care for another person! I was barely caring for my own basic, human needs, and poorly at that. I needed an escape, so I called Ara. I was back to using sex as a hit of dope to take flight on a journey away from processing my feelings. My negative emotions didn't get the proper or respected attention they deserved. Instead, they received a blanketing solution of alcohol and sex.

I had reached a boiling point after Zieya left, knowing she was frail and lifeless when I last saw her. It caused me so much pain that I erupted through the rash decision to climb on top of my roof and slit my wrists. Leo and I had gotten into a fight earlier that day about the elusive Stacy since he went through my phone and figured out that who I had been talking to wasn't a chick. All I could do was feel regret for not leaving with Zi. I took to a bottle of vodka and lay on my roof waiting to bleed out when Leo called Carla for reinforcements. Carla arrived at the house and shimmied her way up to meet me with an empty bottle in my hand and a knife by my side. She grabbed her sweater, wrapped each sleeve around my wrists, and held me while I cried.

Once I stopped wailing, Carla gave me a stern talk about how I needed to start living for myself and quit trying to be with everyone else. In a single second, something clicked in me that craved being alone. I had to be alone; I had to get away. I needed to move to a different state. I wasn't aware at the time that running from my problems was a way to pretend to get it together, that there would be problems anywhere I went since I was the problem. Someone in the rooms of NA once told me wherever I go, there I am; so I needed to quit running and work on myself from the inside, out. Oh, how I wished upon a fucking star that I knew that back then. So, I climbed down from my depressive attempt to kill myself, again, and searched for the map my dad had given me of the U.S. as my childhood room decor.

Closing my eyes and choosing a destination to run away was exactly what I did before I bought a one-way plane ticket to Daytona Beach, Florida. Before I packed my suitcases, I knew I had to tie up loose ends. I told Leo he could stay at the house and I took my name off the lease.

I had to let Ara know that I was leaving. Leo was stunned, but happy I was going to go "find myself" and wanted to show how much he loved me by supporting my decision. The day before my flight, I had a runway show to model some jewelry made by a local artist for some extra cash. I was going to need it since I couldn't pack Leo in my suitcase to take care of my finacial needs. My mom arranged to come to town to see the show and see me off to the airport with sweet goodbyes and fingers crossed that I would make good decisions. I couldn't leave Fanta Se without getting in one last night with my Latin lover, Ara.

Ara had no idea about all the events that were unfolding behind the scenes and was just thrilled to see me again. We smushed ourselves together on his bed and I told him I was leaving. He sat up and protested with anger. He asked me why I was going and why I waited until the last minute to tell him. I was leaving for the airport the next day. I explained how I was going through a rough time in my life and it was time to move on. He knew I wanted to explore more career options with my modeling, so I used that as my main reason for why I was leaving. I couldn't tell him the truth if I wanted him to continue to look at me the way he did, with such adoration and wonderstruckness. I wanted to leave with the impression that I was a good girl who could have been "the one".

I began to get dressed when Ara fell to his knees and hugged my bare torso with his head drooped between his shoulders. I looked down at him and heard his tears fall loudly as if they were those popper firecrackers you threw at your siblings on the Fourth of July. I lifted his chin and asked him what was wrong as the glistening of his face caught my attention. I had never seen such a wholesome expression from a man. I'd provoked men to cry before, but it was never outside of my harsh words. Ara pleaded with me not to go and put up a solid argument for why I should just stay and live with him, but I knew I couldn't. I really did want some respite from the mayhem I felt on the inside.

For a split second, I considered letting myself fall for Ara and forgetting I had ever moved in with Leo. I could possibly be monogamous with Ara and settle down for once. He was, by far, the most amazing lover I had been with at that point, as if his sexual performance was what made the cut for my life-changing decisions. The feeling I got seeing Ara crying over me, begging me, and expressing his longing for me to stay was nothing short of arousing. I wanted him to want me, and there was a whole new level of appreciation I felt he was displaying. Still, I had to leave and stay the course. I had to get out.

I landed in Daytona Beach, FL ready to start my life as someone completely different. No reputation, no ill will done here, just organically, fresh living with new people and a new attitude. My first day on the beach was spent thinking about how I wanted to be happy. So what better place than by the ocean? My thought process was rudely interrupted by intrusive thoughts about my body as I looked at the women around me in their bikinis. The relationship I had with my body and its appearance had always been touch-and-go. I developed an eating disorder as a young teen that stuck with me all the way into my 20s. I was about to be 21, and I was living with a serious case of body dysmorphia. I couldn't ignore the aesthetic that was swarming all over Daytona. I wanted to keep up. I limited my eating even more and started drinking only low-calorie alcohol. No beer. I shared a beachfront condo with a hottie I met on Craigslist, and since he thought I was a hottie, he let me stay there rent-free until I got a job. No, I didn't sleep with Colby as trade to live in his lap of luxury if that's what you're thinking. I simply couldn't resist passing up a chance to hook up with someone sexy that wanted nothing more than to fawn over me; plus, I'm sure he knew I was going to sleep with him since we sex addicts can spot each other.

I had been working as a camgirl to make money, which Colby helped with since he was one of the creators of the site. Camgirls are women who get paid to entertain people behind their webcams on the internet. It's usually a sexually derived profession, but I got creative with it. I sat in front of my laptop, chatting with men who paid me money for my time. Some days, I would just get ready for the day in front of the camera. Others, I would eat a banana wearing nothing but a g-string. It was a means to an end, easy money, so I could afford the life I wanted to live. My priorities were going out to nightclubs, eating out at my favorite restaurants, and shopping anywhere I wanted. Part of being an addict consists of turning anything into an addiction: money, clothes, food, porn. You name it, I was addicted to it. Including power and I felt the power I held by teaming up with Colby.

Colby became somewhat of a manager and confidant who taught me the ropes of how to juggle my power as a female. He was one of the kindest men I had ever met and I felt so seen when I was with him. It's miraculous that he respected me and didn't just skin my body and dump me somewhere since I naively went to Florida blindfolded after meeting him on Craigslist. Colby was five years older than me and had become my best friend. He knew about the shitshow I left behind in NM but didn't know that I couldn't quit any of my men, cold turkey, like I thought I could. I didn't realize I couldn't quit when I got a phone call from Leo frantically explaining an altercation that took place between him and some of his old buddies from high school. What I had gathered was that Leo was drinking at a party when one of his friends made a comment about me being a bitch and a hoe. Not wrong. But then, Leo told the dude to watch his mouth because that was the woman he was in love with he was calling a bitch and hoe. The dude started to talk shit to Leo about him being a dumbass for loving me. Leo then took a baseball bat to the dude's car, which happened to be an expensive race car, and now there was revenge to be had. Leo then told me that the dude's name was Clay Wilson, Randal Wilson's little brother (the guy I lost my virginity to). Fuck! I hate small towns!

The urgency Leo expressed was unlike him. It was unusual for him to show fear, so I was thrown off by why he turned to me for help. I immediately felt like I could save him. I always loved an opportunity to feel like I was needed and I could be a savior, something only men were allowed to portray so it felt like I had the upper hand. I told Leo that once everyone sobered up, a resolution could be had if he just apologized and told Clay that he would pay for the damage. I scoffed at Leo but was flattered since he defended my name and clearly still had feelings for me. It was common for the males I was involved with to encounter violence over me; I thought it was just another form of archaic flattery. Leo then told me that it went deeper than just the car getting wrecked and stated how he now had a hit out on him.

"What do you mean a hit out on you? Like, someone is going to kill you?"

"Yes."

"What else did you do Leo? Why is it extreme enough for someone to try to kill you?"

"M.K. please, I can't explain over the phone, you'll just have to trust me. I love you and I need your help."

I took every word he said seriously and made up my mind to help him. I hung up and told Colby that I wanted a friend to come out to Daytona and live with me for a while. Colby was expecting some cute girl or some gay guy and, without question, gave me the green light. I called Leo back and told him that he could come out and within hours, Leo was driving 1,726 miles to come live with me. Give or take a mile.

Chapter 8

#letsplayagame#8yearstreak

Leo arrived in Florida after driving all the way through with no sleep, snorting lines of who knows what to keep himself awake and only stopping to piss. It didn't take long after seeing him again for me to fall into those buff arms and tongue at that famed lip ring. I did my best to play it cool like I wasn't Leo's ex-girlfriend around Colby, but he knew the minute I introduced Leo as my "friend," that he had been inside of me before. Men have a keen sense for that sort of thing. Friends don't typically sleep together but that rule didn't apply to me. Colby and Leo had a cocktail and hit it off relatively well. It was obvious that Leo was going to be rooming with me so Colby gave me one rule: you have to pay more for his share. Rightfully so, however, I did not have enough money to afford my living on top of Leo's share. I had to pull together some money, and quick, if I wanted Leo to stay. It was later that night that I came up with a plan while out bar hopping with the boys. I had been greasing myself up for this moment—the moment I'd become a stripper.

While the boys were bonding over beers, I excused myself to scope out a well-rated strip club according to the internet. I walked in to see gorgeous women wearing outfits similar to what I would go raving in, doing impressive pole tricks. I thought to myself, " I can do that." I had never seen such a sleek strip club before and I had only been to one other strip club so there wasn't much to compare to. I walked out of the club and reunited with the two drunk men bromancing over their shared taste for exotic dancers when they saw me walk out of the club, smiling. They raised their eyebrows at me as I rolled my eyes at them, playfully suggesting how I would revel in my decision to become a stripper at that club. They both looked me, mouths agape, surprised about my newly found confidence to dance naked (as if I didn't already enjoy doing that), and said "Do it!" like two nerdy fanboys. You would have thought they practiced that with how well executed it was. I had been prepping to perform naked with all the private belly dancing sessions I gave people when I was a teen, what could possibly be so different about strip dancing?

The next day, I went into the club ready to audition when the manager of the club gave me the go-ahead just by scanning my body, as if I was some grocery store item being rung up for bagging. Dare he ask paper or plastic? Anyway, I listened to his terms and conditions for working at the club and he told me I could go in for work later that night. It was Monday and I didn't think there would be much traffic for a weekday, so I agreed since I wanted to practice before the weekend. I rushed home to tell the boys and we all took a field trip to a store that sold exotic dance wear. I was buying slinky outfits and trying on 6-inch stilettos to go with each two-piece, themed outfit. Leo and Colby had their fun dressing me up like a doll as if they missed out on being able to do it as boys growing up forced to play with trucks instead of Barbies. Perhaps it was just them excited to see my sexy body in gear, specifically to arouse men.

It was almost 9 PM and I had to check in at the club at 9:30 PM. I told the boys I wanted them to stay behind my first night so I didn't get nervous and fall on my face. I wasted no time introducing myself to some of the women in hopes of making a friend to cling to. Most of the women had been dancing at that club for years and I knew I would face some criticism for being the new girl. It was time to choose the music I wanted to dance to so I walked up to the DJ booth before walking to the main stage. Gigantic screens behind me played the music video as I slowly walked towards a row of men and women hoping it would distract them from noticing it was my first time.

As each song began to play, a new dancer would take the stage when her name was announced. "Next to the stage is _____!" I had to come up with a stage name and quick and so I told the DJ the first name that came to mind—Zieya. The DJ announced, "Zieya to the main stage," and I walked out ever so gently with one foot in front of the other and thought to myself how all those modeling classes would pay off at that moment. The thousands of dollars spent for the agency I was affiliated with would lead to my debut as an uprising STRIPPER! If only I could have let my mom and the company know how much money I made, I'd thank them.

I walked to a pole closest to where I saw people sitting and remembered I didn't know any pole tricks or how to even climb a pole; most definitely not with sweaty hands and my nerves shaking my spine. It was time to decide how I would captivate my audience with no real "stripper" moves, so I slowly slid down the pole, with it behind me, and sat on the stage while lip-syncing Rob Zombie's "Living Dead Girl". I rolled around, flipped my hair, and gave people the look I would give Leo when I wanted something. No sooner did the song start than it ended with me in the same position I began with by gripping the pole behind me. I improvised my own music video in the form of a tantrum and it worked. I once was told by another dancer that she knew she didn't have to work hard or climb a pole because the money was on the ground, not the ceiling.

After my first round of tips, I knew I didn't have to try hard to get what I wanted and make serious money. A high roller spotted me on stage and invited me to sit with him and his party for a drink. I could tell he was a high roller by his shoes and his watch. I had a special eye for Movados and unique stitching on shoes since my dad had expensive taste. It didn't take long before my charismatic personality won over Mr. High Roller and got me a payday of $1,200 for 10 minutes of my time. It was as if he turned into a horse, eating sugar cubes out of the palm of my hand. With my witts and facetious manner, I got a loyal customer to enjoy my gig of naked acting. It always amazed me to witness how men melted at the thought of being loved or desired by an attractive woman. I knew my goofy and strange behavior was infectious but my appeal, I learned, wasn't just with my body or my face, but in how I would resort to childlike play without placing boundaries on my imagination. Alcohol would also enhance that vivid play. I was a therapist for hurt and sexually deprived men. Seemed I was cut out for this sort of thing given my track record.

It was 2 AM and I had paid my house fee to the manager and walked out of the club with $2k that night. I got home and the boys were up playing Mortal Kombat on the X-box. They made a pact that they wouldn't sleep until they beat the game, never mind waiting up for me. I told them both how much I made with my nose in the air and they both clapped as if I had just earned some noble award. I felt proud to have made money that was going to contribute to more than just myself. It felt good to have copious amounts of money to control, but at what cost? I wasn't bothered that it was by using my naked body or objectifying my sexuality. What bothered me was my ignorance of it all. I wasn't able to comprehend the consequences of making money that way and it began to shape me into someone I would later have to heal. Just like with the camgirl gig, I felt like it was a "have to" instead of a "want to". Thinking, "I have to make money quick and I'm good enough to use my looks for it," rather than applying for a job where my looks weren't a prerequisite for hiring.

I didn't believe I had the credentials for a normal job like working as a receptionist at a doctor's office or a teller at a bank, since doing math in my head wasn't my strongest skill. We all know I had issues with my math class. I didn't understand that I was settling for *fast* and *practical.* I thought I was more valuable than working a job at a fast food restaurant, but failed to put forth effort to work at anything that didn't involve my looks. It was a weird trap. My attitude around making a career choice was shitty and the sense of entitlement I felt just because I had an attractive body and face only led me to believe I shouldn't have to work too hard. I would have had to have some humility to make my first step, but a cocky attitude fit better than slow and steady to win the race I was in. I wasn't ready to earn anything in a disciplined light, but wanted everything in the shadows. The power struggle between money and beauty was one I would fight with for the next 10 years. I did everything to drag my love affairs along with me for the ride. Why wouldn't they follow? I was footing the bill and giving them exciting sex - the dimensions were too easy not to manipulate. I began to enjoy the role reversal of being the breadwinner in my relationships; instead of being the one in need of saving, I was the one saving.

Leo got used to me taking care of him for a change and was relishing in all the free time and comfort, knowing how much I was grossing monthly. I wanted Leo to start working but that didn't happen before I grew to feel resentment towards him, thus giving me an excuse to reach out to Ara. There was a double standard I held over Leo. Give me all your time, but work hard, not too hard, so I can stay on top. Leo finally landed a job as a mechanic but his attitude of inadequacy is what turned me off the most. It was always due to some quarrel with a lover that I would end up seeking attention from another love interest, regardless of my level of commitment. My addiction always took over. Think of it as a safety net. I had received text messages from Ara here and there but never felt compelled to reply with all that I had going on. Having an excuse on deck was what I did best and whatever I told Ara, I knew, would be enough for him to listen. I finally responded to Ara after months of ignoring him and he was overjoyed to finally hear from me. We spent an evening catching up while Colby and Leo were preoccupied with one another. Ara would eventually tell me that he still loved me and he had been missing me more and more now that he and Carla were hanging out. He nonchalantly expressed how she reminded him of me.

I perked up when he shared the news that Carla had moved up the street from where he was living and that they had been partying together lately. It was unusual for me to get jealous since I was pretty open to sharing love and people, but when Ara admitted that he and Carla were getting close, I felt like she was moving in on someone I had chalked up to be mine. I had no idea what my intentions were when I left Ara behind, but I felt like as long as he kept fawning over me, that was all I needed. If Carla was going to take my place, then I would lose any chance of being able to run back to Ara if I wanted to. Keeping people on standby was the ultimate cushion for me to land on, not if, but when, I would fall. And I was about to faceplant.

I didn't want to ask Ara if he had slept with Carla yet because I felt it wasn't my place, and it would also showcase my vulnerability of how much I cared. I started to talk to Ara more and more and after 11 months passed, I connected with Ara stronger than I had with Leo. I wanted to run from Leo and have Ara waiting for me with his arms wide open. Ara filled my mind with delightful hypotheticals no different than I did to others when I wanted what I wanted. The unhealthy and extreme lengths people go to just to feel love and fulfill their strongest desires, to me, is the premise of addiction. I was willing to trample all over anyone for any reason if it meant I was going to feel "good" in the moment. I would promote violence and risk getting in trouble with the law if it meant I could walk away with being right in an argument and that's exactly what happened when Leo and I were fighting all the time and living without any compromises, more so forced agreement. He ended up in jail over throwing a glass at me, hitting the wall behind me, while I destroyed his laptop. I was no peach when it came to fighting but I felt poised that it was him going to jail over me, so I had that "one-upper" mentality. "You do this, watch me do that," and 10/10 times I would outdo my opponent. Until I was forced to stop. Revenge goes both ways.

Leo and I would always make up with intense sex that included our renewed devotion to each other's character defects. I began to pick up on our pattern and I desperately wanted out. I had already jumped states in an attempt to run from my lovers, how could I possibly let go of Leo after becoming more addicted to him? It was when I noticed that my attraction for him started to expire over his failure to meet my expectations that I decided to ditch him in FL and fly back to NM to see Ara. I had just turned 21 and was daydreaming about joining the bar scene back home when I finally got my chance. The day I landed, all my friends, including

Carla, met me downtown at a club to celebrate my arrival. I was truly happy to see her until I got the weirdest sensation in my stomach after I hugged her. She felt stiff and disingenuous judging by the recoil of her hug. I was on guard and told myself that maybe we had drifted apart, and now she was just a girl I used to know instead of my best friend. Carla was always referred to as the knock-off version of me, which I never understood until she would inevitably stab me in the back. I would be forced to see how she had been trying hard to impersonate me. Until then, I let Carla buy me a drink as we stood between the bar and the dance floor when I saw her lips open to tell me something.

I couldn't make out what she said over the blaring music, so I motioned her to meet me outside. She swayed a little too far to the left, catching herself on the door before I helped her onto a bench outside. I laughed at her and asked how much she had to drink before meeting up with me. She declared not nearly enough to sleep with Ara again. Just like that. Carla blurts out how she slept with Ara and began to make fun of his penis, how he wasn't circumcised, and it was too small for her liking. I felt a burn in my throat that wasn't rum this time, full of nothing other than the feeling of betrayal. Carla had known about Ara being my secret lover before I moved to FL and how I was falling in love with him right before I came back home to NM…and she slept with him anyway? I knew that I was the one who jumped ship and left but it's not like she wasn't up to speed with what was going on in my love life. I made it known how much Ara meant to me and I wasn't going to let her betrayal stop me from pursuing him.

I kept my cool by chiming in on the fun and related with her by saying "I know right?" when I thought the exact opposite. The sex I had with Ara was enough for me to fly across the country to have it, again. I didn't want Carla to know what my true feelings were, so I fought through the tears that wanted to form under my eyelids and took another shot of rum. I was about to meet up with Ara after leaving the bar, but I was conflicted about whether or not I should. The last thing I wanted was for him to spot how aloof I was after finding out what he did. He screwed my best friend, never mind how many people I have hurt with who I've slept with, it was about ME. It was time to decide when my phone rang - it was him.

I answered it and the first thing he said was "Hey there sexy lady, I'm tripping on mushrooms and I want to see you!" I can't lie, I was turned off, but I didn't want to miss a chance to scold him about Carla. We all know how much I love an occasion that calls for punishment. I told him "Can't wait!" and proceeded to give him a place to meet me at. I had one of my friends drive me to the address I gave Ara, which happened to be my dad's address!

While I was in FL, my dad and I were in touch again, and I had actually planned on spending the autumn holidays with him. Since we were in contact again, that meant I finally wanted to introduce him to my Mexican lover. I told my dad that I was going to have Ara come over so he could meet him. Little did Ara know that he was meeting me at my dad's house. He pulled up to my dad's new, two-story house that he ended up moving into after he left Patty for her best friend, Shiela. Let's take a moment to dissect my dad's situation, shall we? So, before I left for FL, my dad had cheated on Patty numerous times, only to get a woman who was only three years older than me pregnant. They had the baby before he decided to settle down with Shiela, whom he had known for years, because Shiela was the wife of one of his best friends from the police force. Apple doesn't fall far from the tree, huh? So Ara got out of his car and stared up at the large, white, stuccoed house and asked me "Where are we?" with dilated pupils.

I hugged his psilocybin-induced body and reconnected my eyes with his. Oh, how I missed those green eyes and long eyelashes. I held his hand and eagerly pulled him towards the front door, telling him it was my dad's place and that he was going to meet him. Ara pulled his hand away from mine and froze right at the welcome mat. I turned around to see the most attractive man looking like he was going to hurl. I giggled and told him that everything was going to be fine, and he took a deep breath and walked into the house. My dad had been watching TV while my new stepbrothers were playing pool in the game room. I didn't care for Shiela, so I gave her my classic passive-aggressive hello. Shiela didn't like me either so our conversations were always minimal. I brought Ara to the living room where my dad was and introduced them to each other. My dad stood and gripped Ara's hand as if it was forced respect before a UFC main event. Ara shook his hand and that was the start of me making my way in to be Ara's girlfriend.

I walked Ara to his car and told him I was going to be flying to visit family in Houston for Thanksgiving, but I would be back soon and had planned on getting a place to rent. He offered for me to stay with him and his friends until I found a place, so I didn't have to live with my dad. I told him I'd think about it as if I hadn't already made up my mind. Before we leaned into each other for a kiss goodbye, I wedged in the question:

"When were you going to mention you and Carla hooking up?"

"That was just a drunken night. I don't even remember it."

"You remember that it happened. That's good enough for me. Why not tell me? You know she's my best friend."

"I didn't think it mattered. I was missing you so much, and she reminds me of you. I started drinking and was talking about you with her and it just sort of happened."

"I'm glad a conversation about me can get you both in the mood."

"M.K. stop. You know you are who I want."

Ara pulled me in, kissed me, and growled in my ear as if I was his lioness and he was the lion. It's sexy shit like that that got me in the position to do whatever he wanted me to. Even though I believed Ara when he told me I was who he wanted to be with, I wouldn't just let it slide. I had to get even.

I knew I felt strongly about Ara enough to forgive him, but I hated feeling second best. Even though Ara restlessly expressed how it was me he wanted to date, I couldn't help but feel like I wasn't his ultimate. This was new for me - jealousy this strong. I had a one-night stand with a model on a connecting flight before I landed in NM and felt like that secret was enough to keep my hurt feelings at bay. It was my secret to keep, and knowing I had this secret somehow made me feel good, as if it were a stash of self-confidence I would need on a rainy day. The responsibility I placed on sex to make me feel like I mattered was how I functioned as a sex and love addict. What's the difference? Sex and Love can exist without the other but not for long. There are a few people I know who have waited until marriage to finally have sex with their partner, but that was as if seeing an elephant in the city. To love without sex is what I wished I could have taught myself before unleashing my pain and passion through sex. Pain is equivalent to passion and passion breeds love. You can have sex without being in love, but that doesn't mean a piece of you isn't left behind with that person. The transaction of both love and sex comes at the cost of emotional stability or instability, and all I ever knew was that love and sex were tools and toys, not acts of respect or treasures to keep close to my heart.

I started to unpack my bags in Ara's room and felt that packing and unpacking was now a trend of mine. Only 11 months in FL and who knew how long I'd be living in this place? This place I thought was suitable enough for Ara and me to begin our lives together with a fresh start until he gave me the grand tour and showed me the second level of this beautiful, stuccoed home. I had no idea what drug-making looked like until Ara hollered at some guy who looked as if he had just snorted floating particles from the air as we opened the door. I saw a scale with mounds of white powder and baggies the size of my thumb layed out on a table. I knew I was putting myself in harm's way but didn't want to show any fear. The guy responded to Ara by turning off the stove and greeting him with a unique handshake. I was living in a trap house.

Just like having unprotected sex, I prayed and hoped for the best. That was the kind of love Ara and I shared. Exhilarating and outrageous love. We went up and down with our lifestyle as bad-boy Mexican running drugs out of his home and daughter of a police officer and local model making good by keeping face to protect my last name as much as possible. I didn't want to disrupt Ara's lifestyle choice so I embraced it in hopes of earning his love. My insecurities mixed with his, over drugs and alcohol, were always a way to summon our demons to come out and play with each other. One night, Ara finds some of my modeling prints I had stashed under his bed of me and another guy and began to rage with harmful remarks about me being a stripper and a slut. He screamed in my face how I needed to pack my shit and get out of his house. Once I quit screaming back in his face, I decided to call Mitch (the guy who had felt me up at church camp), since we were now friends and he happened to be an MMA fighter, to come help me. What better flex than to have another guy on standby to come intimidate your boyfriend? Mitch and his friends rolled up in his truck within minutes only to catch Ara running after me to grab me and throw me over his shoulder in the middle of the street. Mitch jumped out of his truck with his friends following him and yelled at Ara "PUT HER DOWN!" Ara was caught off guard and put me down just in time to have 1, 2, and 3 blows to his face by three different men. He knew he was in trouble and all I could do was run to Mitch's truck and leap in through one of the doors they left open.

I watched all three men red rover Ara's ass to the ground for 30 seconds before running back to the truck. I look back through the rear window to see Ara struggling to pick himself up off the pavement. I felt both terribly sorry and pissed off that it took me having to use my power to put him in his place. It was clear at the time that I stood on the grounds of women doing absolutely anything they needed to to defend themselves from a man no matter how vile behavior. I was not going to tolerate physical abuse from anyone, especially Ara and I was hoping he got the memo after Mitch showed up. Mitch took me back to his place right before the sun came up and let me clean myself up in his bathroom. I had never hooked up with Mitch even though the implication was there and he was a good-looking man. His smile alone had me hooked, but there was always something that came between us, preventing us from hooking up.I came out of his bathroom and sat next to him on the couch to tell him what happened.

I remember thinking that if I wanted to hook up with Mitch, now was the time to do it. Woe is me and I need penial comfort. After I was done telling Mitch my story he wiped the tears off my cheeks and I suddenly had this flashback to when we were teens and he felt me up at church camp. All this time had gone by and I still never mentioned that moment he did that. I wanted to, but I was afraid to offend him after all he just did for me. I thanked him for coming to help me and had no plans to criticize the violence he brought with him. I asked Mitch to take me back so I could start moving out of Ara's place and when I got there, I saw a minela envelope on the doorstep with my name on it. I opened it up to find a CD with the words "my heart belongs to you" written in red sharpie. No name, and nothing else on it. I placed the CD back in the envelope and breathed a sigh before walking in the front door. I was amazed that I still had my key on me. I walked in to see Ara passed out in front of the fireplace on the floor. The fire was still going. I can see the swollen cheekbone and remnants of blood from his nose on his shirt. I crept to the back room to see all my stuff already in my suitcases with the analog photos of me and the male model sitting on top. What a slap in the face to remind me why I was in this mess…but let's be real, It wasn't the photographs that did this.

I rolled my luggage towards the front door when Ara was awakened by the dragging of the wheels. He lifted his head and dramatically gave me a head shake of disbelief that I could have let that happen to him. I told him I left the key on the counter and he stood up to limp his bruised body towards me only to say "Don't go." The tears were flowing and my need to help clean him up was how I ended up back in his bed licking the dry blood from his lips. I really can't help but get sucked back into the scene of movies I obsessed over as a young girl.

This is love. Love is getting your ass kicked. Love is flexing on your partner with your band of followers. Love is sexual jealousy only to put you in your place. All the things I thought love was were the very thing that destroyed my soul with no healing in sight.

The break-up/make-up ritual for me was always better each time around. Something about passionate fighting kept me always going back for more. As I'm lying in bed while Ara is showering, I can't help but think about who could have left me that envelope. How does this person know I live here? I did my best to sneak away to listen to the CD in the only other place that had a CD player in the house, the drug room. I heard the first few seconds of a guitar riff and I knew instantly it was Leo. He was back in town. He clearly still wants me to know that he loves me after all I did. My heart throbbed with pain for a bit at the thought of how I left Leo behind in FL. Am I that cold-hearted to have no remorse for the way things ended? I had no time to grieve my breakups with how fast I moved on. I wished I did so I didn't have to mourn them all at once. Processing big emotions wasn't part of my itinerary and I was caught in Ara's gravitational pull. All I wanted was to stay with one guy for a while. I can't juggle them again. Or could I?

Ara called my name and I ejected the CD as fast as I could and tucked it under my shirt between my braw and my skin. I tip-toed out of the white room and shouted back at Ara to let him know I was coming. I twirled the idea of contacting Leo around my finger before biting down on it and stopping myself from pushing send on the lengthy text I wrote. It seemed after the horrific incident with Ara getting jumped that we were closer than ever and I didn't want to jeopardize our new start. I love a restart button. It scares me, looking back, how natural this thought process was for me, to start over like nothing happened with not the slightest acknowledgment of the destruction in my life.

I was a mad woman. Ara was a madman. We were two immature, highly sexual alcoholics who could not function in a healthy manner. I was obsessed with him and him with me. It always took a police report and some jail time, for them of course, before I would finally throw in my own towel and search for love elsewhere. Between our fights and cheating on Ara, I began to feel like our relationship was irrelevant. I didn't want to address my own issues for why we could not function without alcohol so I did what I always did and resorted back to love that seemed more efficient. Every time I would make or break a relationship, it sparked the same high you get when you buy something new. Even though I had run through Leo and he wasn't "new" per se, the time apart made it feel new every time we reunited. I would feel something similar with my dad. I called Leo one night after feeling defeated in the game I was playing with Ara and there he was, on my front doorstep, ready to rescue me. I would go back and forth with Leo and Ara before getting caught one night when Leo followed me to a bar where I was meeting Ara. I had told Leo I was going to meet up with some friends at a bar and when I pulled into the parking lot, Ara was waiting for me ready to hop in my car. After he planted his lips on mine, I looked over his shoulder as he pulled away from my face only to see Leo, tapping on the glass of the passenger side window with the most sinister smile. I had been caught.

Ara turned his head to meet eyes with Leo for the first time and turned back to look at me to ask, "Who's that?" All I could hear was my heart pounding through my veins as if my pulse was a band of bassoons.

Leo said, "Really, M.K.?" as I watched his mouth move in slow motion before I stepped out of the car. I was beside myself and couldn't speak. I walked around to face Leo as his 6 '1 stature sized me down while Ara got out of the car and asked us if there was a problem. Leo decided to extend his hand and introduce himself as my boyfriend of three years, and as Ara shook his hand he replied with a "Funny, me too."

It isn't physically possible to stare at two sets of eyes, let alone one set, without feeling cross-eyed, so in my panic, I started walking towards the door and pivoted away from where they were standing. I muttered to them both "I'm going to go get a drink, I'll leave you two at it," and walked inside. Once I was inside, I sat at the bar and held back every tear that wanted to leak from my face. My friend Joe was bartending and he always knew when I needed a drink. A free drink. Joe asked me what was wrong and I shamelessly replied "You don't want to know."

Neither of my men walked in to join me so I was left to drink by myself. My misery was so familiar and comfortable at this point that I couldn't help but pile on every bad thought, every bad thing that had ever happened to me in that single moment of despair. It was never simple for me to pick apart what my issue was in real-time, but compiling my issues made for better loathing. I knew Leo was done with me. I heard through a reliable source that the two left together and ended up bonding over a joint talking about how ruthless I was and how they share the same taste in a female succubus that screams their name perfectly in bed. I was glad I could bring two broken-hearted men together while I did my best to conceal my broken heart over them. I know I was to blame, but that wasn't something I was willing to live with. I'm never the bad guy, just a shell of a person doing what I know to do. Getting attached to a person was the easy part, being forced to let go was where I felt death approaching. I would feel suicidal every time I had to detach myself from my love affairs. I had to lay low with some friends before finding a new place to live since I was exposed for cheating on these men with the other and it was only when Leo refused to be in contact with me that I able to break free from the love I had with him. It's when push comes to shove that I am forced to let go.

I knew nothing good was going to come from trying to repair my relationship with Ara. It didn't stop me from trying because we ended up working things out briefly before he started to punish me for what I did with various forms of physical and emotional abuse. I spent countless nights crying over Ara until I finally felt strong enough to break free from him. The only way to do that was to move, again. It was time to hit the other coast after my stay in FL and head for CA. All these years of living a double life just to keep up with my lovers had me wanting a carefree, beach-bum lifestyle. Plus, Zieya was there. I had wondered what she was up to and what was going on in her life sign I lost touch with her. I had no plan when I got to San Diego other than to stay away from relationships.

I found a spot to rent, that my dad of course co-signed for since I couldn't stay in one place long enough to accumulate a respectable rental history, and began to look for work. It took all of three weeks before I landed on the idea of quick money again, and what better way to attain that than with exotic dancing? I told you I was a creature of habit. Since I am so predictable, I'm sure you can guess that I started talking to Leo again and he eventually met me out in SD. I never learned my lesson and I was ok with being a repeated offender while everyone else around me was biting their nails with fear of what was going to happen next. What happened next was drug dealing at the strip club and what I thought was a foolproof system. Leo was by my side as the dealer in the club and I drew in the customers. Leo and I had been turned on by each others' bad boy/bad girl personas even though I knew we were a ticking time bomb. That was the way we liked it. One of the dancers at the club became my best friend and told me about this dancing abroad gig that she wanted me to do with her. It entailed me going with her to her home island of Guam where we would dance on a three-month contract. The club provided lodging and guaranteed money. BIG money. I was so money-hungry that I was willing to do anything to get my share of what I thought was freedom. The island is a U.S. territory so I felt safer going there than if I were going somewhere south of the San Diego Border. Plus, the island was filled to the brim with military personnel due to the Marine, Naval, and Air Force bases out there. I wasn't about to turn down being surrounded by sexy men in uniform.

I broke the news to Leo that I was going on a stripper business trip (I can't even say that with a straight face) and told him it was the perfect chance to make enough money to buy him a new truck and possibly put a down payment on a house when I got back. I was feeding him pictures of a happy, cozy life as if I were holding flashcards and teaching him what he didn't already know. I knew Leo wanted a life with me and my broken promises were how I go him to agree to let me go. It was a week later that I hopped on a flight with Jocelyn to her home island of Guam. Just seven hours later, I was on a tiny island in the middle of the Pacific Ocean, ready to have the summer of a lifetime! Would you be shocked if I told you I had no intention of staying with Leo? I placed myself in a position, yet again, to do my best to secure love with Leo and live my life as a free agent. None of it would work out in the end when I got the news that a funeral was being planned.

It had been weeks of utter sexiness. Sexy men and women, sexy food, sexy atmosphere; this island had a strip that reminded me of Las

Vegas and I was making easy money by being a tease. I felt like I was on top of the world as I stared out over the horizon looking through my Fendi sunglasses. I was doing well for myself but struggling to keep Leo at the forefront of my mind. I was talking to him every day through Facebook Messenger since that was my only means of communicating, keeping him in the loop every chance I got. But, that began to fade the more I faded. I was a lush, no doubt, and liquor helped me with the long hours of pretending to be interested in conversions with people who were my meal ticket. Nothing mattered to me when the booze took over my mind. I was invincible and impenetrable to people's opinions of me. Let's just say the kind of confidence I had when I was drinking was as if I had red lipstick smeared on my teeth and was still able to pull Tyler Lockwood from *Vampire Diaries* to come and wipe my tooth clean for me. Foolish, I know, but it was working for me. I was flirting with everyone around me, including a fellow dancer.

I knew I wanted to sleep with her but I had to break it off with Leo first. I was trying not to cheat this time around so I could somehow be a person of substance over style. I really was trying to better myself, but couldn't help but get trapped in the wake of my sex addiction. When I got off my shift early that morning, I went home to Skype Leo to break up with him. I was honest with him, something I'd never done before, about how I was attracted to this Columbian woman and did my best to let him down slowly. I knew I wasn't ready to settle down and I think Leo knew it too, but we both wanted me to be ready to quit being so wild and free and be more domesticated and docile. As I made my claim, he responded with tears and shutting down. Just like my father's silence towards me, I expected Leo to shut me out, even after I extended the "let's still be friends" bit. He blocked me on all social media accounts, and since I didn't have an active phone number, there was no way to reach him. I thought that he was for sure out of my life this time.

We hung up the Skype call and that was that. I was done trying to be with Leo and I wanted to discover more of what I was capable of doing, such as how much money I could make and who I was going to fall in love with next. My life's premise was to fall in love with a new person! I was an addict on the loose and no one was around to save me from myself. I felt like I had been living my dream of being an independent woman with no shame around my job or how many sex partners I had, ready to take on the world as a liberated Latina. I wasn't going to take shit from anyone anymore about the way I was living! What better place to gloat about my wreckless lifestyle than FB? It was when I was checking all my comments from pictures I had posted that I saw I had a message from one of my friends from middle school.

Hey M.K.,

It's Maximo. I want you to know that Leo is in the hospital from a suicide attempt. His mom flew out to SD to be with him and your old neighbor at the apartment complex was the one to find him in a pool of blood in the bathtub. He severed his tendons that connect at the elbow and doesn't have mobility in his arms right now. I'll keep you updated on his condition. I know he blocked you but he wanted me to show you the damage so here's the picture. Hope you know everyone blames you.

Later, Maximo

As I clicked on the small tile that indicated the attached picture, my throat grew dry and my face felt like it was already pale in color.

The picture enhanced as I zoomed in to see Leo's arm and all the blood that flowed down into the tub. It was a dangerous amount of blood from what I saw and I began to fret at the sight of his wound. An adult human body can lose 5-6 pints of blood before it dies and I'd say Leo was right at 4 and a half. With my hands covering my face, I let out a scream so loud that I lost my voice. I stayed up crying for hours and didn't know how to cope with what I saw other than to drink. I responded to Maximo's message by letting him know a little bit of my side of the story as if I owed him or anyone else an explanation. I didn't want to be blamed for what Leo had done to himself so I asked Maximo to give Leo a message from me asking Leo to unblock me so we could talk. I told Maximo to let him know that I was sorry and that I loved him. I really did love Leo, but not the way Leo loved me. I never heard back from Maximo and Leo kept me blocked so I was forced to move on with what I knew as fact; Leo was back in CA in bad condition and I was stuck on an island feeling like everyone hated me. Leo was the victim and I was the slut who broke his heart. I was so over all the slut shaming. I wasn't sure how to process my emotions other than to just keep running. I had planned to continue my travels by going to Japan next and then New Zealand after that to forget about the horrific events in my life. Then I met a gentleman named Isaac.

I hadn't felt a love like Isaac's since Zieya. Isaac was hard to beam in on. I recall him telling me he didn't want to hook up with me the night we met, which surprised me since we ended up skinny-dipping in the ocean. Isaac was the first guy to tell me that he didn't want to have sex with me while I was drunk so I could make the decision based on free will rather than sloppy drunkness. I was impressed and he won me over. I hadn't believed I deserved any kind of chivalry or respect for that matter. Ara, Leo, Christian, and even the women I dated hadn't really given me a perspective of what I should mean to myself over what I meant to them. Zieya was the first person to help me notice my self-worth and now Isaac was helping me sober up and see that there was more to me than a party. He helped me sober up and I will always respect him for that. A clean-cut Air Force boy was just what I needed. Just when I began to trust in my ability to stay sober I got a message from Zieya. It read:

M.K.,

I miss you. I heard what happened to Leo and I think it's tragic that you guys ended the way you did. Not like I know the details but he is out of the rehab facility and living back in Fanta Se with his mom. I wanted you to know how much it makes me happy to see you are living your best life from all the pictures I see on FB. I'm living my best life too. I got married and had a baby! I know it's been too long since we last spoke but I am still so in love with you. If I could just make you mine I would want to run away with you and raise this baby together and live out our lives like we were supposed to all along. I love you M.K. You will always be my greatest love.

-Zieya

I read the message and felt my ego wanting to celebrate by bragging with thoughts of "of course, I'm her greatest love, everyone tells me that" when I quickly interrupted that ripple from taking over with a knock on my door. It was Isaac. I was glad he interrupted me because I didn't know how to respond to Zieya's message. I was in a weird place of wanting to feel remorse, but knowing how desired I was kept me on a high horse of pretentiousness. I didn't want to know anything about anyone's life and staying self-consumed was how I was surviving. What would I even say to Zieya? "Thanks for noticing my wreckless lifestyle, I love you too?" Like?? I can't do anything about the way I felt towards her, I knew that, but I was across the globe preparing myself to be with Isaac. I was relieved to hear that Leo was recovering and that he went back home to be supported by the wretch of a mother he has. Lord knows I have to forgive her every day for the role she was about to take in my life.

Chapter 9

#deathshroud#thereveal

I was up to my head with being a material girl and was parading around the sexiest interracial relationship I'd ever seen. Isaac's blue eyes and night sky skin had me wanting a proposal real quick, but I knew there was no way that would happen with how things were going. I had thought I had everything that I wanted, everything that would satisfy my craving for living the highlife, but no dice. I started to spend money on body modifications to ease the craving of wanting more of something, but not knowing what that something was. It became a ritual to schedule appointments at a local tattoo shop to have my skin sliced open for dermal piercings and sit under the needle for my longest tattoo session yet. It was my version of therapy as the dopamine released the euphoric feeling of both pain and pleasure. I always felt more beautiful knowing I was covering up who I really was with each sparkly gem pulling attention away from the flaws I saw on my body. It was no different with my tattoos, each explaining a story of the pain I went through in the form of a beautiful art piece.

Every time things got heated between Isaac and me, I would go sit through a session at the shop and think about each stage of our relationship. We were at the stage of opening up about our pasts when Isaac disclosed to me that he was still in love with his ex-girlfriend from back home and I admitted the trouble I had caused over my alcohol addiction. Things didn't seem too reassuring for our future. I was aware enough to know that drinking played a huge role in my life, but I had never admitted to a significant other like I did with Isaac. Isaac was forthcoming about his porn addiction and shared his fantasies with me in hopes to draw us closer and I was honest with him about my sexual cravings with both men and women; all my kinks and secret pleasures around sex. Naturally, he was the match and I was the kerosene. One thing I noticed about shacking up with another sex addict was the fight that had always been resolved with sex. There was no amount of sex that could keep me with Isaac after I was forced to leave the island, for good.

Isaac and I had been at odds with each other the day I went and got the most elaborate chest piece of my tattoo career. I was on my back in a deep meditative state as each stroke of the tattoo machine scraped my skin with tribal black ink when I felt my phone buzz under my butt. Without moving my torso, I gingerly moved my hand to reach for my phone from my back pocket. As I pulled my hand up above my face I saw the famous red circle of IOS notifications on top of my FB app, I grappled with the idea of whether or not I should check it. I wanted to wait to open it so I didn't mess up the tattoo artist's steady hand but my obsessive compulsiveness never let me shrug off a notification. I opened up Messenger and saw 'Kristi Gonzales' at the top of my messages. My mom took my stepdad's name and was no longer Reyes. I hated that. I lit up and was eager to read a message from her since it had been weeks since I last checked in with her. It's hard to keep a clear voice lying to my mom about what I'd been up to. I tapped the thread and began reading.

> Hi honey,
>
> It is with a heavy heart that I share that Zieya has passed away. Her body was found at her brother's apartment here in Fanta Se. She committed suicide M.K. We can't believe she is gone. Please call me when you can. I love you so much.

The saliva in my mouth suddenly dried up and I felt like I was choking. I stared up at the ceiling, and with the calmest voice, asked the artist to take a break after lying underneath his hand for the last seven hours.

He responded with an "I was wondering when you were going to ask" and released his elbow from locking me in place, allowing me to sit up. I wasn't sure if I was experiencing the pain of my raw skin exposed to the air or the pain of getting the news that the only person who saw me for me, loved me for me, was dead. With each inhale I felt a pain firing off in every direction of my body as if my insides were a circuit board and someone just poured water over it, only to watch it spark and malfunction. I found enough energy to balance myself on my feet and walked to the bathroom where I looked in the mirror and told myself that it wasn't true. The lie I told myself was how I was able to walk out of the shop and call Isaac. I sat on a rock stone wall facing the ocean while I waited for Isaac to show up and let out a scream so loud that I felt the waves scream back.

Isaac arrived in his car and couldn't make out what I was saying since I was still sobbing when he showed up. He helped me into the car and did his best to comfort me by letting me have a conniption while he gripped his steering wheel in discomfort. You know the awkwardness of people not knowing how to react to people crying and falling apart? The look of confusion and uneasiness while emotion is being shed? That was Isaac. I punched his dashboard until my knuckles started to bleed and as we sat in idle, the fumes from the car began to strangle me so I told him to drive. I stuck my head out the window and took a deep breath while the wind stripped my tears from my face. I was silent the whole drive home before sharing the news I received from my mom. Isaac didn't know the whole story about Zieya; only that she was my stepsister and someone I didn't talk about much. He leaned in to hug me, but couldn't fully embrace me since I had plasma leaking from the thick layers of ink on my chest. He drove me home and comforted me any way I would let him. For the next 24 hours, I drank myself into a deep sleep, forgetting about any attempt at sobering up and leaving the option to self-medicate with alcohol behind me.

It was time to call my mom and hear what she knew about what happened. I wasn't given much information and it drove me crazy. Every question I had about how she died was met only with visceral answers. To my mom's knowledge, Zieya had hung herself in her brother's closet after being in town visiting family. I asked where her baby was and where her husband was. My mom deflected from all of my questioning with her own projection of worry and concern for me. I felt a tone of paranoia in her voice and I knew exactly what she was thinking. Why wouldn't she have that thought? I had been troubled by my mental health my whole life. I could use this to be the perfect excuse to take my own life. As much as I wished I had the gall to pull the plug on myself, I could never bring myself to do it.

The pernicious effect of losing her meant it was time to catch a flight home. I scanned through flights online and the soonest I could get all the way back to NM was five days out. The funeral was taking place a day before I was scheduled to land and there was nothing I could do about it. My anger began to take over and I was annoyed, anxious, and heartbroken. What was I going to do about Isaac? Was this the end for him and me? I waited until he got off work to have a talk about what was next for us, but until then, I did what I always do...reach out to what's familiar and comfortable to cope. My comfort had two looks at the time, Leo and Ara. Leo had already traveled across the country, both ways, for me, why would he finally decide to show up on my doorstep in the condition he was in this time? Ara had been in contact with me through email since we weren't friends on FB, due to all the blocking that took place, but it was very brief. I knew he wanted to keep me at arm's length so I had to take a back seat with using these men to get me through my negative emotions. Or would I?

I composed an email to Ara asking him if he would be willing to video-chat with me so I could share some unnerving news with him and within hours I got a reply. He agreed to meet with me over Skype and the second his pixelated face popped up on my screen, I felt a sense of calm and relief I hadn't felt since finding out about Zieya's death. Why was Ara's availability for me the answer to my panic? I wasn't in a position to figure that out at the time; all I knew was I wasn't going to let him slip through the cracks of my fingers, again. I wanted nothing more than to have him hold me and make everything better. The amount of pressure I placed on my lovers, even my family members, to make me feel better was unrealistic. I had no clue that my own peace was something only I could unlock and Ara would place this same kind of responsibility on me. During our call, Ara told me that he started doing heroin after we separated, and I couldn't help but blame myself and want to save him. I found out later that his elaborate tale of being addicted to one of the most dangerous drugs was a lie that he used to reel me back into his life. I wasn't the only one who knew how to fish.

I landed in NM and instead of going straight to my mom or my dad's house to grieve the loss of my "stepsister" I went straight to a concert where I had a VIP pass given to me by the guitarist Brian Welch from the band Korn, who surprisingly wrote a book about becoming a Christian himself. But not before we met on the connecting flight from LA to NM and planned to party hard. I wasn't about to pass up an opportunity like this. My priorities were always to have a good time and avert any duty I had that required clear thinking. I wanted everyone to know how much I was affected by Zieya's death but didn't want to display any responsibility or proper gestures to show how much I cared. I know everyone grieves differently: some laugh at funerals and some go to counseling, but I was drinking and partying, and that was what worked for me. Was this typical addict behavior? Get distracted with what was preferred rather than working towards an honorable reputation? Over exaggerate my feelings so that others go unnoticed by my obnoxious behavior? I didn't give two fucks what anyone thought about the way I was handling her loss, or living my life for that matter, I was just doing what I always did. No one knew how much she cared about me and how much I loved her, and I wasn't going to just accept her death until I brought someone down with me.

My second stop was to visit my dad at the police station after I bought myself an Audi TT with the cash I had stashed away from working at the club. I needed a way to drive around town and play Sherlock Holmes to find out more about Zieya's death. Who better to ask than the man who oversaw the officers at the scene? I wouldn't show up empty-handed in hopes of bypassing any heavy questioning my dad had about my personal life, so an Armani watch was just the ticket. Like father, like daughter. I had hoped he'd jumped straight into gratitude for my expensive love gesture and not bring up the question of how I could afford such a gift. It was in his office overlooking our small town's main street that I nonchalantly brought up Zieya's death.

"Did you hear that my stepsister died?"

"Zieya. Yes, I did. It's sad."

"Do you know what happened?"

"I do."

"What happened?"

He told me the officers on sight claimed that she had attempted not once, but twice, to hang herself. The first attempt was with a black trash bag, but it couldn't hold her weight and snapped. The second was with a belt she wrapped around the clothes bar in her brother's closet, and that time it worked. What kind of person is that determined to make it happen? I would have thought it was a sign from God if the bag snapped on me like that. My dad looked at me with a furrowed brow and responded, "A desperate person."

I left his office feeling shaken but still dissatisfied after those gruesome details of her passing. There were still so many unknowns like "Why was she really there in Fanta Se?" and "Where were her son and husband?" As I sped off with the police station in my rearview mirror, I knew I had to settle in at my new living quarters with Ara so I braced myself before showing up to his new place. As I walked to the door, I shifted my attitude to jump back into his life like I had never left and told myself that I was only here for one reason, and that was just to find out what happened to Zieya. Ara answered the door and I was greeted with that same smile and those big eyes that hooked me all those years ago. Here we go again. I walked in after embracing him at the doorway only to get punched in the face with the aroma of Marijuana. Ara quickly introduced me to his roommate who I swore was his doppelganger and I did my best not to stare for too long. I broke away from shaking the attractive man's hand and distracted myself by addressing the elephant in the room. "Are you guys growing pot?" Ara giggled and began to give me the tour of his house, just like old times; he was still where I left him and I was no different.

It took no time before I let my thoughts be consumed with investigating what happened to Zieya. The few leads I had were her brother and his apartment, which happened to be the same apartment complex I lived at with Skarlette. Eerie. I was lying next to Ara while he slept and began thumbing through my FB messages to see who I could contact to ask questions about Zi when I saw an unclicked message dated months ago. That damn blue dot escaped me while the commotion of my party life in Guam took over. I opened the thread and began to read a message from Bryson Wallace, a name I had only heard once before.

Hi M.K.

I know you don't know me but I know you. I've been watching you for a long time and I think you are the most beautiful thing I've ever seen. You were friends with my older sister in middle school and I was a part of your friend circle but we somehow never met. I've always thought you were the perfect girl for me and since I never got a chance to be with you, I started dating your sister. Don't worry, I loved her with everything I had. If you ever want to finally meet, here's my number # 505-555-5555.

I could feel the vomit forming in my stomach ready to make its way up to my mouth. I sat up and went to the living room to text the number and drank a shot of whiskey to help me sleep. Ara always kept brown liquor in the cabinets. I went back to bed and waited for the number to respond to my disarming text of a simple invite to meet up. I wanted to know how this guy ended up dating Zieya and why he was such a douchebag after stalking me for so long. His FB page wasn't much help for clues around Zieya's life before she died. All I gathered was that he was extremely attractive and had two children of his own. Zieya had a husband and a child of her own and was living in CA, or so I thought. How did she end up with this guy? I wanted nothing more than to find out as my eyes grew heavy and it was time to shut it down before the sun came up. I needed to rest before I went stomping around town like a pouting child who was ready to cause a scene.

I woke up that morning to Ara kissing me all over and happy to have me back in his bed, again. I began combing through the bed looking for my phone before telling him good morning. He sensed I was frantic and offered morning sex to calm me down. For once, sex wasn't going to fix this problem. I rebuffed his offer and jumped out of bed to get ready for the day as fast as I could since I got a reply from Bryson. The text read:

Can you meet me tonight?

I replied with a time and place and Bryson agreed. I contacted a friend who managed the only strip club in town and told him I was going to have an important meeting at the club, asking him to keep an eye out for me. It was regime at this point to talk to strange men in strip clubs, so it seemed like the perfect place to interrogate Bryson. Before I could rehearse my questioning, the day had gone by and I was pulling up to the club in an outfit that spoke both "don't try me" and "I'm even prettier in person," ready to get my answers from someone I deemed my enemy.

At first glance, Bryson appeared devilishly handsome with slicked-back, blonde hair and a jawline I wanted to punch. I thought it was the strobe lights that made him so attractive, but as he got closer, I began to blame it on the whole accidental genealogy thing. I didn't want to give him too much credit, but it was hard to ignore that face. He introduced himself and offered to buy me a drink, to break the ice I assumed, when I aggressively answered "no" and got straight to the point. I went down a long line of questioning giving Bryson no room for small talk when he started off by telling me that he was on my side, the good guy as if I were also "the good guy," somehow displaying a noble gesture in getting to the bottom of what happened. I wasn't ready for what he was about to share.

"So Zieya and I met through Leo."

"My ex Leo?'

"Yea. Leo came back to town after rehab and needed somewhere to stay so he hit me up. We go way back."

"I thought he was with his mom?"

"He wanted out from under her watch, understandably. That woman was smothering him and we decided to be roommates until he ended up back in CA right before Zieya died."

"I thought that's where Zieya was, with her husband?"

"She was until they got into a huge fight and her hubby told her to take some time to cool off, he thought that she might have been suffering from postpartum depression. So she came back here to be with family and that's when she hit up Leo since she found out he was here recovering from his broken heart."

"How did Leo introduce you to her?"

"He didn't, I just sort of stole her from him."

"WHAT?!"

Bryson continued to tell me that Zieya ended up meeting Leo at their house one night so they could support each other over how much I sucked and how much they resented me. Zieya felt bad for Leo after he shared his suicidal story with her. Bryson proceeded to tell me that Leo and Zi ended up sleeping with each other and after that happened, Zieya was always around. Bryson noticed Zieya noticing him and they eventually started connecting, ultimately choosing Bryson over Leo and that set Leo off. Apparently, Zieya went snooping through Bryson's laptop one night with a clear view of the FB message he sent me and read his weird stalker love note to me. After Zieya read the message, she ended up moving out and going to stay with her brother, and that's when Leo decided to take matters into his own hands. Bryson stopped talking for a few seconds to sip his vodka tonic and fiddled with the cocktail straw before continuing.

"Leo found Zieya's husband on FB and called him to tell him that he had slept with his wife and that she was out here hoeing it up. That she needed help and he thought he should know because if it were his wife, he'd want to know if she was screwing around on him."

"No he fucking didn't! That bastard!"

"Dude called her up, asking her about the affair, and threatened to take full custody of their son. He told her he wanted a divorce and she killed herself the next day."

"How do you know all of this?"

"Leo. I was upset that I pissed her off by sending that message to you. Maybe if she would have just stayed with me at my place, she'd still be alive. I was going to kick Leo out anyway since she and I talked about starting a life together, but once he realized she chose me over him, he left willingly. He couldn't stand being second best."

"Nobody can. I'll be in touch."

It took every iota of strength within me to walk away from Bryson without going off in a spell of rage ending with me crying on the ground. I walked outside to my car holding back an identical scream like I did when I first found out in Guam. Once I locked myself in my front seat, I let it rip. Leo? Zieya? I couldn't comprehend the magnitude of what I was just told, but I felt it. I felt the icy sharp blades of pain that would lead to my revenge. I wanted to call Leo, but I couldn't. I was still blocked. I wanted to scream at Zieya, but I couldn't. I wanted to punch Bryson in the face, which I could have done, but I didn't. It was late and I needed to go home to Ara and take my aggression out on him in the bedroom. I needed a hit of my favorite drug.

I hadn't planned my next meeting with Bryson since I was still processing everything he shared with me. We began to text each other more and more, sharing our stories of chaos with previous lovers and that's when I added in that I was seeing Ara. Bryson didn't care if I was taken, he finally had me right where he wanted me and he wasn't going to let me go. It had been a couple of days since I saw Bryson last and I decided to invite him over while Ara was out for the day. I was going to just sit with Bryson in his decked-out, red Xtera and talk to him, but when he drove up I felt compelled to invite him inside. I didn't feel he was a threat, but someone who was soft and kind like I was, deep down. As I shut the front door behind him, I knew our meeting was going to go differently than expected.

"I'm sorry if the way I let you in on everything was too much. I just wanted to tell you the truth."

"Thank you for telling me the truth. That's all I wanted."

"I loved her ya know. She was amazing. I was ready to move her and her son in with me and blend our families together."

"Why did you message me on FB, Bryson?"

"Initially, I was drunk and jealous of Leo. I hated the back and forth she was playing with us."

"I wonder where she got that from?"

"Then I realized that she was just like you in so many ways. Or a different version of you. I know this sounds crazy, but I had been wanting a chance to cross paths with you. And here I am! In the most fucked up way."

"You don't even know me."

"I know that I'm here now, and so are you. I'm just like you M.K. Desperate and looking for love."

I started to cry when Bryson reached over to tuck my hair behind my ear and leaned in to hug me. I was so certain that this stalker frat boy was just another asshole waiting to ruin someone else's life, similar to what I did to my lovers, but then he started to cry. I looked him in his eyes and the glassy blue reflection filled my body with warmth and an urge to embrace him back. I should have known better than to get lost in his eyes - it's my kryptonite. I let him hug my limp body when I straightened my spine and closed my eyes so I didn't act on impulse. My desire to kiss him reverberated with him falling into me for a kiss. My excuse for allowing him to kiss me was irrelevant; after all of what I had known to be fact, I wanted nothing more than to just exist in that moment. Our heavy kiss led to our naked bodies on the couch for less than five minutes. Bryson got off of me and said nothing besides "I'm sorry" as he dressed himself and I sat in familiar disappointment, but thinking that I had got what I wanted which was some weird satisfaction of knowing he had slept with Zieya and I felt close to her while he was on top of me. Sure, I granted Bryson's wish, but it was more about Zieya for me than anything.

I assured him that it was fine that our sex wasn't some daytime marathon and that I was used to it. Stamina on the first go around wasn't something that was practiced by the men I slept with. There was a sense of training that always took place after I agreed to enter into a steady sex life with some of them. Bryson left and I cleaned myself up before Ara got home. I wasn't worried about Ara suspecting a thing since I had the cheating on my lover act down. It wasn't much for me to keep a secret but I started to feel the side effects of spiritual sickness. You know the kind of icky feeling that makes you want to crawl out of your own skin? Add that on top of feeling woozy every morning and cradling my bruised skin from Ara grabbing me during his drunken episodes. I had known I was pregnant before I peed on a stick, but I had to be certain so I made an appointment at Planned Parenthood after I skipped my period.

I hadn't been in touch with Bryson after our excerpt of sex on the couch and was racked knowing Ara and I had been having unprotected sex for years and I hadn't missed a single period. Was Ara sterile? It's not like I was diligent about taking my birth control over the course of our sex lives together, so why now? I felt it in my bones that it wasn't Ara's kid. It felt as if I had no other choice but to tell Ara it was his. After my urine test and blood work came back positive for an eight-week pregnancy, I knew it was time to tell Ara. My plan was to tell him that we couldn't afford to have a child right now but promised him I would give him children one day if he agreed to abort it. I thought about how I could hide the abortion from him until the doctor explained what the procedure would be like. I had never had an abortion before and the pain and discomfort I experienced was something I had never wanted to go through again. Passing a fetus through my body after taking an oral treatment made the next 24 hours of my life miserable.

Bed rest and Tylenol were how I survived the trauma of an abortion. I threw in some alcohol to make sure I could sleep after witnessing all the blood I left behind on the couch; the very place this all started. I crawled to the bathroom in hopes of making it to the shower but the pain was too fierce. Ara was out walking the dogs so I called him to come help me and he ran home and lifted me into the shower. I was so confused why this man was so good to me in moments of despair, but when it came to our drunken escapades, he would torture me. Maybe I was constantly getting back at him through all the secrets I kept from him. My thoughts were running wild as I cleansed the blood running down my thighs and told myself it was time to call Bryson and lament over this fucked up scenario.

I woke up the next day and texted Bryson asking him to call me. He never did. He ignored all my texts, forcing me to leave him a gnarly voicemail describing what I went through, and no sooner than I hung up the phone, I was getting a call back. Bryson didn't second guess my assumption of him being the father since he had been down this road before and knew how fertile he was. I took responsibility for my end, I just wanted him and I to talk about this since it was necessary for me to move on from my mistake. He asked me if he could pay for half of the cost of the procedure when I told him I just wanted to meet up with him to talk about everything. We met later that day and sat at a table at a coffee shop this time, and I pleaded with him about how this needed to stay between us. Bryson handed me a wad of cash and insisted he pay for the abortion; I could tell he had done this before. I looked at Bryson and said, "Promise me B; promise you and I are good and we take this to the grave." Bryson put his hand on top of mine, smiled a smile of contempt, and replied "I promise."

Chapter 10

#predictable#sickbride

I never understood that being sought after and lusted over by people willing to ruin their marriages or lives wasn't the ultimate measure of worthiness or of how desirable I could be. I thought that if someone wanted to have sex with me, they would love me and I would finally be accepted, perhaps even cherished. That wasn't the case, but like I said, I never knew that. Although sex can be sacred and used to grow closer to the person you love and to show love, sex itself is NOT love without the intention of respect. I barely had any self-respect so I wasn't prone to showing anyone else the respect they deserved. Ara and I ended things for a final time after we reached another breaking point when word got out about Bryson and me sleeping with each other. I'll never really know how Ara found out, but what I do know is that the truth always surfaces. After the stunt I pulled by lying to Ara about him being the father, it was made known that things weren't repairable after that. He deserved more respect than I had to give, as did I, and it was time for me to leave Fanta Se behind me and keep my distance from every guy in it. I found myself bound for San Diego yet again. Old habits die hard, right?

I moved to Ocean Beach and was living life sober for the first time since I started drinking at 13. It was so liberating for me to be sober and single. No abusive relationships and no booze to help clear my head for the next 8 months. I didn't think I was capable of doing it, but I accomplished that time with the help of the beach and slowing down long enough to fall in love with myself and discover strengths I never knew I had. It was hard to stay away from promiscuous sex because, let's face it, sexual cravings are impatient, but I did give myself rules about starting relationships out of my encounters. It was difficult not to be noticed with all the modeling I was doing and the recognition I was getting when I would go out downtown with my friends, especially on the eve of my birthday. No matter how important I felt or how cool the scene was, I refused to pick up a glass.

I had always found the term " too much of anything can kill ya" as an over exaggeration to keep people from having a good time, or feeling good until I fell prey to this very concept. I'd known firsthand that too much sex and alcohol could cause trouble and the trouble I had caused in my life thus far was never lived down. I had always been given a heap of shit for being someone who was never involved enough or consistent in one particular thing, but in my defense, I always felt like I was balanced with everything I chose to pursue in life. A little bit of everything to *start* and *stop* whenever I pleased, just to keep life fresh and exciting. I was definitely consistent with my erratic behavior. As each day passed and my mind began to awaken from the numbness of the alcohol, my emotional and physical body began to come to the center and I had to sit in the aftermath of my exhaustion of constantly starting something new. I wanted some relief from myself and all the cravings I was having so I broke down in tears and began to pray.

I didn't know how to pray in a way that I thought was "appropriate".

I wasn't even sure whom I was praying to! One night in my room I began to speak as if Zieya was in the room and her spirit was surrounding me, letting me know I was safe, so I spoke soft words in what I thought was the form of a prayer. I had always recited prayers that were forced by memorization as a child, but never intentional words that came from my heart. When I was younger, I witnessed my dad pray over meals and my mom pray over our road trips, but I was never taught that I had the power of prayer within me. I don't remember ever having anyone lay hands over me in prayer or anyone explaining to me the importance of prayer for my life, but I wanted to take my own interpretation of prayer and try it on for size. I didn't believe that God wanted me to be his follower, whatever or whoever God was, so I placed Zieya in front of all my spiritual speaking. It seemed to work since I was feeling better than I had ever felt! I was able to taste a sliver of what it was like to be healthy on the inside and that promoted healthiness for other areas as well.

Who would have thought having a spiritual side would be so renewing? I was reading more and more and eating healthier to keep my new lifestyle intact. I began journaling some of my heavy emotions and got real with myself about my eating disorder. I had even made some new friends who weren't negative influences on me and wanted to get to know me on an intellectual level. It seemed like I was set for success until my past resurfaced with a single phone call from Leo. After two years of not speaking, Leo and I got to have a conversation at last. I looked down at my phone from an unknown caller and answered with a chipper *hello.* On the other end was a deep, yet smooth voice that stated "Hi, M.K." and my mouth fell open at the sound of his voice. I didn't know what to do! Should I hang up? Should I go off on him?! Do I immediately start apologizing for how things went down?!

So many thoughts zig-zagged before I answered with the calmest voice saying, "Hi back, Leo."

There were tears flowing and lots of apologizing after our two-hour-long conversation revealing our intentions behind our actions over the entirety of our relationship. That also included Zieya. I acted as if it were the first time I heard anything about him and Zieya when he began to share his side of the story. The whole time I was listening to him portray himself as a martyr I felt my subconscious kick into revenge mode. The blood in my veins began to pump faster and harder as I listened to him explain his reasoning behind everything and all I could do was tune him out long enough to hear the ringing in my ears. There would be no way to tell if I were upset if I just gave him a fake, kind, response and that's exactly what I did. Any remorse I had, or feeling of missing Leo had gone away the moment I was triggered by reliving the news of Zieya's death. What I really wanted was to explode with hurtful words and tell him to go slit his wrists this time, but instead, I took a deep breath and plotted in my head how I was going to get him back by playing nice. This was a marathon, not a sprint and if I was going to avenge Zieya, I would have to approach this carefully.

Just because I sobered up for eight months didn't mean I became a good person. I was still as cold and manipulative as ever, but this time I was going to be the queen on the chessboard. I told Leo that we should meet up if he felt like taking a break from his girlfriend he had been with for the last 11 months. I had planned to go to a rave at the Hard Rock downtown over the weekend and invited Leo to come. Benni Benassi was in town and I knew Leo couldn't resist since Benni was our jam throughout our relationship. I set him up with the perfect temptation and was excited to watch him squirm as he grappled with making a decision. I made it easy for him to decide by letting him watch me decorate my skin and strap my body into the flashiest outfit over a FaceTime call. I hadn't been drinking, but I felt like a relapse was in order since I was going to see Leo in a matter of hours when he quickly got off the phone with me and said he was going to get ready to come with me. Phase 1 was complete. I got Leo to agree to see me and what better condition than half-naked, covered in gold glitter? He was on his way over and it was time for me to take that shot of liquid courage. I couldn't stomach him sober. My roommates were already in the kitchen pregaming for their night and with one fell swoop, my eight months had been down the hatch.

Leo showed up at the house in his girlfriend's car as I stood at the front door, towering over a staircase leading to the street. He looked up at me like he hadn't ever seen me before. A look that implied I was new to him. I looked back down at him and his hand was on the hood of the car as if it were preventing him from falling over when I noticed I was slightly drooling over how good he looked. Damn. I hate it when that happens! The guy you so badly want to hate is so good-looking that it makes you not want to hate him! Leo ran up each step to greet me at the top of the stairway. With each of us standing on the same slab of concrete staring at each other, I was thrown off by who should make the first move. Before I could initiate a hug he rammed me up against my screen door with a hug, lifting me in the air and kissing me. The move was slick and as I looked down at his face, I thought of every time I had been in this exact position looking down on a man, in more than one way. I wrapped my legs around him to keep myself supported and hugged him tight. I can't lie and say I didn't enjoy it. As he put me down I asked him if he was ready to roll and he responded with a sassy "I've been ready." I grabbed Leo's hand and we took off in my drop-top with the red leather interior accenting our sexual tension as we cruised down the I-5.

Heavy bass blanketed the top floor of the hotel as we walked into the party and I began to feel the warmth of those tequila shots I took before we left. Leo broke free from me to head to the bar while I slid my way to the front of the dance floor so I could feel the vibrations of the massive speakers on my, already rattling, body. Through a crowd of people sliding off one another, I see a shirtless Leo walking back towards me with his tongue hanging out and as he got closer, the flashing lights helped illuminate a tiny paper square that sat on his tongue, dissolving. I looked at him and shook my head with a smile. I had never done acid so I wasn't sure what he was in for, but I knew that whatever happened, I was blaming it on the drugs. Leo and I wrapped ourselves around each other and let the sweat from our bodies drip like the liquor from my lips. I was sloshed and Leo was out of his mind, or maybe he was finally in tune, whatever it was, it reignited our love. We looked like an M.C. Escher art piece by the time we were done with the night. A rabbit hole of intoxicated sex would lead us down the aisle to say "I do" six months later.

Leading up to our nuptials, we spent countless hours blowing off of each other, mixing liquors to fuel our fights, and hoarding resentments to later use against each other. It was becoming a habit for me to bring up Zieya every time we had a fight, and it goes without saying that I blamed him every time. I would grip my hair and fall to the ground with tears streaming anytime I would cross my threshold with alcohol. No matter how many times Leo would apologize, I would stick my finger in the open wound and turn it. We were stuck on a loop, as usual, and it was over a big fight that I called my dad to grieve my emotions over Leo. I had told my dad I wanted to dump Leo when my dad calmed me down by rationalizing the situation for me to stay in the relationship. It was odd to hear my dad press me about staying in my relationship with Leo, so I knew something was up.

I wouldn't find out what the two men in my life were conspiring until Leo got down on one knee and asked me to marry him during a photoshoot. I will give it to Leo, the proposal was epic but I was livid when I found out that he had been talking to my dad for months, behind my back, and asked my dad for my hand in marriage. So archaic, but I also respected it. It wasn't something I felt flattered over but turned off by since I knew Leo was not my person and my dad was the only man I wanted to work towards. It was uncalled for since we were not in a position to be married. My dad would have known that if he spoke with me like he spoke to my lovers. My dad made it known that he was keeping the friendships he forged with my exes no matter how I felt about it. My feelings really didn't matter to the men in my life, except Jax, and even if I had the qualifications to articulate my feelings to the men in my life, I was still brushed off as a "drama queen." "That's just what M.K. does." It's sickening and I was hurt that I now was stuck between a rock and a hard place. My brother seemed to have been my only friend at the time.

I knew I didn't want to marry Leo, but I said yes in the moment anyway. I liked the idea of marriage, but I knew my polyamorous lifestyle didn't really mesh well with the sacrosanct of married life. Being with one person, or monogamous, is something celestial to me; out of this world, and in no way did I believe a single human could be with another single human for the rest of their life. I know modern day marriages are an array of agreements, but I'm pretty sure Leo was expecting me to keep outsiders out of our marriage. I believed he thought he could make an 'honest' woman out of me and I wanted that for him too, but that was far from what I was willing to give him. As

Leo picked his body up from kneeling in the sad, he jumped right into slipping a customized ring on my slender finger, holding my hand in the air for the photographer to see. I couldn't help but feel a wave of thrill by being freshly engaged and the center of attention as I stood on the beach posing for each click. Nothing ever good came from having that much attention and I've said it before so I'll say it again…my first round of addictive behavior came from all the attention I was given.

First Christian, now Leo, and I had one other half-attempt at a proposal along the way, but I was too self-centered to follow through with it—as if anything had changed. I loved me a man who wanted to marry me, I just didn't love the man who wanted me to marry him. After the high wore off, I felt like I was making a big mistake, but didn't want to say anything much less call it off. It was just days ago that I had slept with one of my photographers and now I was engaged. What was my life? Seriously. I was terrified deep down but kept up with appearances, just as modeling teaches you to do, alongside social media. All the phone calls to relatives and our obnoxious photos of our engagement posted online were enough for me to decide I wanted some comfort from my family. I was done with California living and I knew Leo and I needed to make a change if we were going to break free from some of our tumultuous behavior. He was going to have to stop selling/doing cocaine and I was going to have to stop cheating/bullying him.

The side effects of us being typical addicts included: cutthroat words as fighting amo, sexual aggression, punishing behavior, substance abuse, and possibly but not limited to mental breakdowns causing episodes of rage and abuse. We needed some adults around to help us since we were acting like children who needed supervision. I had already used and abused New Mexico so it was time to head to

Texas. My entire family on my mom's side was there and I felt confident that they would help Leo and me get things on track. It was wishful thinking that pushed Leo and I to pack up our lives up and head out East to start the simple life of small town living. Jax had been with Leo and me out in CA for a couple of weeks visiting before we made the trek back to my hometown and he saw exactly how we were living. It added to my decision to move home and since my brother was my closest supporter, I knew that he would stand by me no matter how this shitshow played out. I look back and regret introducing Jax to my lifestyle, especially with how up close and personal things got because he was about to make some of the very mistakes I was making.

Leo didn't understand that I wanted to do my best to stay sober, and since it had been the culprit to many bad decisions, I suggested that we stop drinking after our engagement party. We invited friends from NM to come to TX for the festivities at my grandparent's estate. We sucked at being a couple, but we sure knew how to party. Leo's mom was one of the guests who arrived from out of town and as you can imagine, she wasn't too happy about our engagement. She never liked me and I respected her decision to not like me. I didn't like me most of the time but I really didn't like her. She was one of those moms who raised her boy as if he were her lover; a surrogate spouse syndrome case which meant she made my life harder than it already was. After our engagement party, I was done drinking and had every intention of having another sober stint. If I could make it 8 months, I was going to anti up and make it a year this time if Leo would just get on board but that was impossible with his mom around.

Tammy was one of those women who constantly needed validation that she was still desirable in her old age with all the plastic surgery and priceless jewelry she had to flaunt. This woman couldn't hang on to a man and was more manic than my hypochondriac grandmother. She was a crystal clear vision of my future if I didn't change the trajectory of my life. You know that notion that the very thing you can't stand in another person is the very thing that you do? That was Tammy for me. Before Tammy left town to go back to her assisted living lifestyle since she pissed away any shot at having a good man to take care of her, she did her best to taunt me by bringing alcohol to our house to drink with Leo one last time. In Leo's eyes, she could do no wrong and vice versa, but I made it clear to Leo that I was done and he should be too. Tammy then started to harass me by saying that Leo was a grown-ass man that could drink if he wanted to so I left the two of them at our new house together feeling betrayed that Leo chose his mom and a bottle of Patron over me.

I did anything and everything to keep myself distracted from drinking, even if that meant drifting from Leo and cheating on him. Jax had made himself comfortable at our house and came over any chance he got and soon became Leo's drinking buddy. Misery loves company, right? Any time I came home after an evening out from sleeping with my side piece or dinner with my family, Jax and Leo were at our dining room table, drinking and doing lines. A freshman in college sulking with my grown fiance was just too gag worthy, especially after finding out they both slept with my friend Meena to get back at me. Jax and Leo deserve each other. I was losing my brother every moment I chose not to drink and felt like Leo wanted nothing to do with me in a sober light. Maybe we don't actually like each other without the substance in full effect. We for sure didn't love each other the way a healthy couple ready to go the distance would. Every time I started over in a new place, in a new home with new hope, I noticed it would always come crashing down the moment a violent outbreak from alcohol was involved.

I thought this time would be different but it wasn't. An eruption of cops left Leo and I surrendering with our hands in the air after drinking one night. I relapsed. It was time to have some peace and guidance in our lives and the only person I thought that could help was none other than Lars. My dad had been in a good place in his life and I was on speaking terms with him so why not let him intervene? Maybe his influence on our lives could whip us into shape and he could provide the adult supervision we so desperately needed. Back to Fanta Se we went. I never imagined going to Fanta Se again. But hey, my life was one giant recycling bin, and I couldn't seem to ever be on the same page with Leo so I was ready to be close to my dad in hopes he could help me squeeze some toothpaste back in the tube.

I found a two-story farmhouse two miles away from where my dad lived and I was excited to be out in the country. The thought of being in the city was too close for comfort with all of the bridges I had burned. I had met up with a selective circle of old friends and was ready to mingle over drinks while Leo was at work. I hadn't been too keen on getting a job since we had just moved back and I felt my duties were to get our home in order and plan our wedding. Giving Leo what he wanted, when he wanted it, was the price I paid to stay home and live my double life. Although I've never had sex for money, I've engaged in sexual acts for the things I wanted out of my lovers. I'm pretty sure that's still a transaction; it's not like I knew that true love didn't keep a tally. Leo was my fiance, so that meant my sex cost him a new car, a big house, and whatever I wanted without argument. This was how I ruled with power and it was only getting worse by mixing in abusive behavior. It seemed that there was no stop in sight especially after I hooked up with Ara one afternoon. He had been day drinking and so had I, so why not? He was going through a break-up and Ara knew I was engaged since he looked at my ring before I straddled him on his couch. We gave no fucks. That's exactly what sorry people do. What addicts do. We don't have a care in the world, no respect for others, and not a hint of acknowledgment for our own choices that eventually lead to destruction.

If you've ever had sex with someone and you know it was going to be the last time, for real, then you know that feeling of fear in being alone. Giving up sex means giving up a false sense of security that we were loved and now won't be loved again. I knew Ara was my false sense of security and I could not keep relying on him to make me feel like I was worth something. I was desperate and it was time to stick to my word and walk away from these sorry situations by staying sober. No more alcohol! On October 31, 2016, I had my last drink and I was prepared to face the worst just to stay clean. That Halloween night I was partying a little too hard and was in need of some care when I got too drunk and ditched by Leo. Who better to care for me than one of the greatest guys of my life?

You know that one guy friend that you have always wondered about but never actually slept with in fear it would make things weird and then you could no longer be friends? That's Guy. Guy Blakely was my lifelong friend I could always count on. He was the one who listened to all my drama stories with boyfriends and took care of me when I was too drunk. Guy was there when I took my last sip of rum before tucking me in bed and making sure no other guys barged into my room to take advantage of me. Before I passed out, I hugged Guy and remembered thinking to myself "Why can't I date nice guys like Guy?" Just as Guy was leaving, Leo came home after storming off over me crying to him about how tired I was from the toxicity of drinking and cheating and I wanted it to stop for good if I was going to say "I do" at the altar. Leo finally saw my heartache over my addictions and agreed to stop with me so the next morning we made an oath to keep our D.O.C. (drug of choice) away from us.

That morning was Sunday, and I woke up from a text from my dad asking me if I wanted to go to church with him and his new family that he managed to weave together after all the time I had been away. It seemed that my dad was on the up and up from being the active predator I knew him to be. My dad told me he was in counseling where he discovered his truth about **exploiting vulnerabilities in different women and preying on their weaknesses, gratifying his need for intimate power. My dad shared with me that once he began to lose interest in these women, he would find himself trying to leave the relationship by preying on another woman.** His cycle sounded all too familiar and I had to give it to my dad for being so candid with me. This kind of honesty helped me make my decision about his offer to go to church so I told him yes. I also wanted to please him since it became my second nature no matter how much blame I was still holding over his head.

I pulled myself together well enough to make a church appearance at some hotel ballroom; that's how new the church was with no permanent building to call home. I didn't mind, the smaller the better so the likeliness of anyone I knew spotting me there wasn't an issue. Not like the shame I walked around with was discrete, why would I care who spotted me in church? Leo however, wouldn't be caught dead at church so he decided to stay behind. My dad was volunteering on the security team so I sat with his new wife Shiela, and their newborn daughter alongside my other half-sister. No wonder this man wanted to go to church, he needed it more than any of us with that line-up. I had been quick to judge him, but the reality was that he had been my only hope at the time.

I went to church that Sunday to please my father but left with an understanding of a heavenly father that I didn't need to please with my performance. I learned that a one-on-one relationship with God was just a decision away, no different than my sobriety, and it got me excited to go back to learn more. I thought only people in prison found Jesus and all other believers were just delusional people claiming to be the next Messiah or falsely proclaiming Christianity for their own self-fulfilling prophecy. There are in fact those people in existence, but it seemed like everyone I met at Sage Church was a straight shooter. The service was quite enjoyable and was nothing like the church I grew up in. Apparently, not all churches are copy and paste, and this church had me curious enough to mimic their beliefs. The only way to learn more was to keep attending and that is exactly what I did. One time turned into three times and three turned into me leading a women's small group with Sage Church. I was so captivated by Pastor Rodney Colt and his deliverance of a spiritual message that I held my steadfast decision to be a Christian with white-knuckle intensity and was ready to take the next step.

Leo couldn't stand to see me turning my life around and smiling all the time so he chose to come to church with me to find out what it was all about. We eventually decided to get baptized after teetering with the concept since we were embarrassed to go up on stage and get dunked in a tub full of water. We were just two hard-core sinners thinking God could never love us for what we've done and now we are standing in a massive church about to make one of the biggest decisions of our spiritual lives. On November 13, 2016, I was baptized as a profound symbol of dying to my old self and picking up my cross to be made new. I believed it and it was everything to me at that moment! The Greek word *baptizo* means to 'immerse' which to me was exactly what happened when I went under and came out feeling washed of anything bad that has ever gone down in my life. I had never experienced anything like it and that night I had a vivid dream about a shark being beached just at arm's length away from me, which Google later translated by defining my dream as an expression of my worries and I was finally safe from my fears. Whatever my dream meant, it was a dream that had stuck with me like no other dream. Aside from the church having an outstanding greeting team, worship music, and non-judgemental church goers, it had outreach programs I eagerly wanted to be a part of, particularly their prison ministry since Jax had been in and out of jail since we left San Diego and it was weighing on my heart with how to help him.

I hadn't been the best example for my brothers for what it was like to live a humble and happy life with no drugs or violence. What Blake and Jax saw was a daughter with a mouth on her and a sister with an attitude to take whatever she wanted, thinking there was never any consequence. Jax was suffering from the consequences by sitting in jail for days at a time until my dad would come around to bail him out or my mom would put up the money for his bonds and Blake was in the beginning stages of an abusive relationship. I so badly wished my brothers would come to church with me to witness my and Leo's newly found faith being put to work, but I got it. It's hard to backtrack and start fresh with a new mind towards church. They were jaded no different than I was, and I couldn't help them unlearn what they had already learned. I had felt judged for so long and so did they. Scripture had been the only tool I believed wasn't intended to judge me and I wanted to share that with others, especially my brothers.

We were steadily going to church and the joy people carried was something I wanted. The church taught me the fundamentals of knowing Christ and making Christ known with the hope that the love I accepted from God would be the very love I could show other people. It felt like the love I wanted to display all along was coming to fruition with how well things had been going with Leo and me. I had kept my promise of staying sober and I hadn't felt any urges to cheat on Leo which resulted in having more time to develop my attraction for him. We were growing on a deeper level of intimacy that didn't involve sex, which was foreign to me. I had never been involved in a relationship with spiritual connection before and I was beginning to think that that was the missing link. It was the day before the wedding when Kourtney came over and pointed out how much weight I had lost. I responded to her with a gleam of excitement because I was just another female who associated my health with how skinny I looked. I had been losing weight more rapidly than usual without starving myself so I couldn't help but think it was all the work I was putting in on the rescue farm I had started.

One of my dreams was to have my own farm of rescue animals, and that was exactly what I did. My dad helped me set up a corral on my 1.5-acre property so I could adopt a horse, two pygmy goats, and three dogs, one of whom was pregnant and gave birth to a litter of nine puppies. I was big on my spiritual connection after finding my church and the farm helped me tap into animal therapy. Taking care of the animals gave me purpose outside my addiction just as the church gave me guidance for caring for life outside of my own. I was hours away from marrying a second guy in my lifetime and I had been feeling woozy. Was it Kourtney's comment that had me pondering my health or was it my anxiety over the wedding that was to take place the following morning? That night, I got this feeling that forced my body to toss and turn with a humming inside that felt like an internal warning sign. I couldn't sleep at all and when it was finally time to get up, I noticed that the feeling stuck with me all the way down the aisle. Maybe it was me being nervous about riding my horse, Ginger, down the aisle to meet Leo at the altar? Or maybe I was getting cold feet? Whatever it was, I could not shake it.

The pressure that my generation underwent to be married with children before we were 30 is formidable. Society had taught us to prepare ourselves to graduate from college and know what career path we wanted before squeezing out a couple of puppies with our high school sweethearts. Conforming was not something I did well and I most assuredly wasn't having children with my first love, much less marry him. I knew I didn't want to marry Leo either, but I wanted to be married to not only comfort the loneliness I felt but also to make my very traditional family, happy. I knew I loved Leo but I also resented him to no end. I blamed him for Zieya's death, but I also took pity on him which made me want to be available for him, but only when I saw fit. I wasn't taught that more than one feeling could exist at the same time so I would incessantly beat myself up for not loving Leo the way I thought he should be loved. Even if I wanted to love him with my all, I was only interested in giving him part of me; the part of me that did believe I was capable of being in this marriage even when there wasn't a piece of paper to legally bind us. I had still been legally married to Christian and hadn't been able to find him to serve him with divorce papers so I just ignored it, like I did with any other problem I had in life. Out of sight, out of mind.

There was one thing I couldn't seem to put on the back burner and that was all the symptoms I began experiencing. It was shortly after our empty vows that I skipped my period and made an appointment to see my doctor to find out what I had been fearing all along. Leo wasn't aware of what I was experiencing with all the fatigue, extreme thirst, or constant tremors that seemed to always take place when I was driving. If you've ever sat anxiously in a waiting room with your leg bouncing up and down without your foot ever leaving the ground, then you know how your mind plays tricks on you to come up with the worst possible scenario. For me, it was being pregnant. The doctor walked through the door and I knew right away that she was going to confirm my pregnancy by the look on her face.

"Ms. Rave, you are about eight weeks pregnant and I put in an order for an ultrasound later this week." I wanted to fall to my knees and scream at the top of my lungs no different from when I found out about Zieya—no different than the last pregnancy. I quietly responded to the doctor by saying "My husband is going to be elated over this news," as she walked out. I felt that my being pregnant was just confirmation that I was going in the direction I asked for.

I went home and did my best to shed my doubts about being a mother to Leo's child and cried so hard it turned to prayer. My relationship with God at that time was shallow and being a new believer, my understanding of God's love was minimal. The idea of a God being omnipresent, omnipotent, and omniscient wasn't for my boxed mind to comprehend. I did my best to hide my real feelings from God and lied through my prayers. I waited for Leo to get home that evening and prepared myself with a fake smile, ready to share the news of my trembling fear of parenthood with him. I wanted him to feel like it was something to be celebrated so I put on my best act and was ready to reassure him that we could do this. I've always loved children, but I told myself I never wanted any of my own. After the suffering of my abortion, I reminded myself that I was never going to go through that again and if I ever got pregnant, I was going to keep it. Maybe this was the right time for me to settle down and have kids and leave my partying behind me, where it belonged. Leo wanted fatherhood and I knew he wanted to have the picture-perfect family he never had.

I made it to my ultrasound appointment with a renewed outlook on how I was going to do my best to grow this baby and let the joy of innocence influence my life in a happy way instead of dreading the process. My optimism would soon be met with a frown from a sonographer while she searched for a heartbeat on the monitor. As I lay on the reclined chair with cold goop on my belly, the nurse left the room to go grab a doctor to double-check her work as if she wasn't confident in her efforts. My worst thought came to life when the doctor explained to me that the fetus was no longer alive. Here I am on my back, again, getting heartbreaking news just like in Guam. My skin grew cold and goosebumps sprouted on my arms as I sat up in the chair. The doctor ordered more blood work and left the room to give me a moment to grieve, alone.

I was sent home after being told that I was about four months pregnant and was going to have to pass the miscarriage the same way I did when I had the abortion.I called Leo to tell him what happened and he rushed home as soon as he could only to walk in on me in a state of hysteria. I ran to him and fell in his arms like I had been doing for years and repeatedly stated I was sorry as if it was my fault the baby didn't survive. Leo held me all night and made the call to our parents to let them know what was going on. It wasn't until the next morning that I received a phone call from my doctor asking me to come in for an appointment to discuss the results of my blood work. I headed to my appointment with my mom by my side after she arrived in town to support me, which was exactly what I needed when the doctor explained that I was on the brink of going into DKA (diabetic ketoacidosis) because I was in fact a Type 1 Diabetic.

I've had alcohol poisoning, OD'd on ecstasy, lost two babies, the love from Zieya, and now this? This was something I could not heal from as the doctor explained my blood glucose levels to me and prescribed medical treatment to help me stay out of the hospital. She explained that I could have gone into a coma if I would have waited any longer. The average adult has a normal blood sugar range between 80-120 and I was told that my bg (blood glucose) level was at 560. It was no wonder why my baby couldn't survive in my body; my blood was toxic and trying to kill me.

For those of you who don't know a damn thing about diabetes, like I didn't, other than a common correlation of sugar and extra body fat, allow me. Type 1 diabetes is an autoimmune disease that CANNOT be cured with any modern day, Western medicine. It can only be managed by using insulin, a synthetic hormone, in lue of a functioning pancreas. The pancreas is an organ in the body that excretes insulin to help blood sugars enter the cells in the body to use as energy, that energy coming from food. It's a vital organ, to say the least. This disease was commonly known as Juvenile Diabetes and the majority of diagnoses were found in young children ages 3- 12, but now it can be found at any age. I was 26 and suddenly told my body was failing to make its own insulin because my body was attacking itself. Type 2 diabetes is when a pancreas makes less insulin thus becoming resistant to making it. I could have just cut back on unhealthy eating and exercised more if I had been diagnosed with Type 2, but no. I was in the category of having no cure and having to identify as a rare type of diabetes known as 1.5 LADA (latent autoimmune disease in adults).

As I sat on top of the medical table, I looked over at my mom and gave her a look that asked her to be my ears for me because I had started to shut down. I relied on her to listen to the doctor's instructions for my new life of medicine, injections, and finger pricks. The room began to close in on me and my vision became blurred. I felt like I was ready to die.

My dad came to meet my mom and me after leaving the hospital and that was a meeting I will never forget. My parents came together to be there for me in a way I never would have imagined. It never occurred to me that turning a new leaf and making better decisions for my life would result in a crippling disease that I would be stuck with until the day I die unless a cure is found. But let's face it, diabetes has been around since the Romans discovered how they had it by drinking their own pee. I was doomed. I had no hope and trying to detox from sugar to get my levels back in an area that wouldn't cause organ failure landed me back at my grandparent's house in Yellow, TX. I was calling 911 so often after my diagnosis because I was having seizures and anxiety with how to dose myself insulin, that my parents decided I needed to be watched 24/7. My mom was more helpful than my dad at the time and she was the one who decided that I should live with my grandparents. My dad found it difficult to be available for me aside from giving me the drill sergeant talk about how I wasn't going to die or let this disease kill me while pointing his fingers in my face. My parents both lacked sensitivity and knowledge toward this sensitive subject and clearly didn't know how to process their own emotions, much less help me process mine over my illness.

The withdrawals I suffered from had me so impaired, that I felt like killing myself, for real this time. The human brain is encased in subdural fluid which is essentially sugar water and when deprived of appropriate levels to function, there is no living life normally. I couldn't sleep, walk, eat, or shower myself. I had been stripped of any amount of dignity I had and reduced to mush it felt like. Or maybe that was just my brain feeling like it was shriveling up and falling out of my ear every time I had low blood sugar. It was the vertigo spells and cold sweats that led to mood swings and feeling drunk when my levels got too high. It never seemed to stop and I couldn't take the torture anymore. A bullet to the head would be my preferred method in taking my life since all the other ways seemed to prolong the pain. Every waking moment that my body was reacting to acclimating to normal blood sugar levels was a moment I felt I couldn't ever come back from. I was ready to go. Take me, God.

I was afraid of food and even more terrified of the spinning sensations I got after I ate. I thought I was done with those nights of laying in my bed drunk with one foot on the ground making sure I wasn't about to fall off the earth, but I guess not. I could not believe that I got sober for this. What did I do to deserve this? Million dollar question, right? Doctors claim it's nothing more than a fluke, that my case was rare and since I didn't have any family history of Type 1 Diabetes, there was no real explanation for what happened. One theory was that my body must have undergone an extreme illness or trauma causing a gene that had been dormant to flip, causing my GAD (glutamic acid decarboxylase), an extra antibody to form. Another theory was from a Shaman who suggested that my pancreas turning against me was directly because I suffered from letting love in. True, but was that really the case? My theory was the brown recluse spider bite I got on my 18th birthday causing me to become paralyzed from the waist down until doctors surgically removed the venom from my back. I heard it was common in South America for people to have developed Type 1 Diabetes after being bitten by one of those suckers. Who knows?

You know what all these theories have in common? Trauma. Evidently, I have had enough trauma in one lifetime that my body had had enough. I thought quitting cold turkey and changing my lifestyle choices would result in a healthy outcome but this was far from healthy. At least in the beginning. Leo had been going back and forth between TX and NM to visit me which took a toll on our intimacy so I decided to move back home to be with him. At that point, I had been slowly adjusting to my new lifestyle of medicine and was coping by acting out in extremes. My mental state had been suffering when I decided to shave my head like I was Natalie Portman in *"V" for Vendetta*. Luckily my head was nice and round so I was able to pull it off and Leo was still attracted to me, but that didn't mean I felt secure. I was the most insecure I had ever been and to top it off, Leo and I had been discussing our future attempt at a family when I told Leo that I was done trying to have kids. The fighting began to frequent and I had done my best to not blame God for why I got sick but instead to turn to Him for my sanity. I started to pull away from both Leo and my faith when I decided to reach out to someone else. But who? I had given up Ara and I wasn't interested in going backwards anymore. I needed something new.

Instagram. Oh, how those DMs have gotten me in trouble. No amount of marriage counseling could have saved Leo's opinion of me after he caught me talking to another guy by scrolling through my iWatch since I deleted the threads on my iPhone. Such an inconvenience on Apple's part to make me delete two separate threads. Leo had made up his mind that I could not be forgiven and wanted to split; saying divorce was too official since we weren't legally married.

However, in NM there is such thing as common law marriage and that meant we would have to agree to share everything we had purchased together, and if we didn't, it was warranted for court. That was exactly what I was prepared to do since I wanted everything. I told Leo that if he really wanted to split, I was going to keep the house, the farm, and the car.

Leo had stolen my car in the middle of the night after he moved his stuff out of the house, which was painful to watch only because it was one of my exes who helped him. I felt a sense of relief as he was loading up each box but I was confused as to why I was fighting so dirty. Was it just something I learned to do by watching my parents? Was it all revenge? Or was it my defensive mechanism to protect my very real feelings of being abandoned? I didn't love him enough to treat him the way he deserved but I didn't want him to leave me either. I wanted to seem like the victim since he was the one who ended things and I was just the one who made the mistake. I thought being Christian meant you forgive and move on with your marriage but I see why Leo couldn't take my abuse any longer. I was a hot mess and cheating on him was enough for him to defend himself. I had been doing it for so long that he couldn't/wouldn't tolerate it any longer and taking my car was his way of telling me to "fuck off." But I couldn't let Leo leave thinking he had the last laugh, so I called Jared.

Jared had been a hot-shot lawyer in Fanta Se and famous as my dad's rival. He and my dad used to be on the police force together and while Jared went his way, my dad went his. I'm not sure about the whole story for why Jared and Lars ended up hating each other, but I had known that this guy watched me blossom into a thorned rose since he had been a part of my life, my whole life. Jared had been lurking in the weeds ready to shake my pedals and I knew it. Time to play innocent M.K. and make the phone call that got me what I wanted—Leo to return my car and scared shitless so he knows not to ever fuck with me again. Jared's number had been saved in my phone after he and I saw each other out in the wild when he handed me his card with a grin implying I could give him a call after hours. I knew how to abuse an offer, that's for sure, and if you ever offer one, I'll take two. So I called Jared to tell him my story and he came over within minutes of hanging up.

Jared walked through my front door with a sleek suit on that smelt expensive enough for me to extort. I thought he was sexy for his age and I hadn't known any 40-something-year-old lawyers who had full-sleeve tattoos and kept themselves fit. I knew exactly what was about to go down, but I made sure he knew he was in my back pocket at my disposal if we went through with hooking up. Jared wasn't a sexually deprived man who wanted so desperately to be desired by a young hot thing. I knew it was just me whom he wanted to conquer. I can spot my own kind. I had secretly always wanted to know what it was like to sleep with an older man since my particular brand of sex usually came my age or younger. I knew he was going to get my car back, but I also knew I wanted to feel adored since Leo left. I can attest to campaigning for the concept of "the only way to get over someone is to get under someone else." So after our terms and conditions, it was time to sign on the dotted line. I knew Jared was married with kids and I knew how powerful he was, but most importantly I knew he wanted to bend me over my couch. This wasn't the first time Jared cheated on his wife and this wasn't my first rodeo with using people as my drug. Jared was my lowest point when it came to my sex addiction, the equivalent of using public toilet water to line your syringe before you shoot up with heroin. I felt like not even God could help me out of this one.

Jared left my house with instructions for me to retrieve my car once he found out where it was and before you know it, I was back on track to being a functioning addict. I couldn't cave to alcoholism since my diagnosis scared the shit out of me, so texting men and looking for love was my only vice left. After Zieya died, I gave up trying to pursue women so it was just a single, clean-cut man I was after. I had everything I fought dirty for: my car, house, and freedom, so I was feeling perky about bringing home my next suitor. Loneliness had been my greatest fear and the only thing that helped calm my nerves was to have someone around. It didn't necessarily mean I needed sex from that someone; I just needed them to exist where I was. My dad and stepmom knew I was going through a lot and couldn't find the time to be available for me emotionally so they tried to help by sending my stepbrother, Brad, over to check on me. Brad is six years younger than me and was the troublemaker of my stepbrothers. He was the bad boy who always brought home a different girl to our family gatherings and tried so hard to be cool. These characteristics run deep in our family even though we aren't related.

Brad showed up and I was in bed upstairs when I heard his footsteps climbing to greet me. He walked over to my bed and sat down next to me and asked how I was doing. It was sweet to see Brad show an interest in my well-being even though he had been the stepbrother I knew nothing about, nothing that mattered anyway. I started to cry and told Brad how melancholy I was over all the drama that was going down when he slipped in a gentle "Want me to hold you?" while I was still talking. I quit ranting and sat up to clear my throat to ask him to repeat himself.

"Do you want me to get in bed with you and hold you?"

"Brad, you're my brother."

"Stepbrother."

"Thanks, but no thanks."

"I just thought it would be nice to comfort you, plus what happened on New Year's that one time."

"Brad, nothing happened on New Year's Eve. You are crazy for thinking that we could be anything other than stepsiblings."

"Fine, I'll go."

I pulled the covers over my head and screamed into my pillow after Brad walked out of the house. As if my life wasn't complicated enough, I had my stepbrother trying to move in on me after he reminisced on a time when he thought I had hit on him while drunk at a New Year's party. I vaguely remember that night all those years ago, but what I do remember is my stepbrother flirting with me and complimenting me every chance he got only to ask me to be his kiss at midnight. I'm sure I flirted back and made fun of him for thinking I was hot, but I knew for certain I didn't kiss Brad at midnight because I kissed someone else. Not sure who, but it wasn't Brad! I do know that Brad had always stared at me every time we were around each other because I would catch him and his intense gaze by looking back at him and asking him "What?" in a teasing manner. I thought it was harmless but really it led to some deep-seated feelings for Brad leaving him with edging emotions.

After Brad left I couldn't believe how I had potentially led my stepbrother on in a way that would insinuate my wanting to sleep with him. I knew sleeping with stepsiblings was a thing but the last stepsibling I slept with killed herself so I was not going to go down that road again. I realized I needed to clean up my act and was starting to recognize how sick I was mentally and emotionally, not just physically. I had always been trying to prove that I was worthy by performing to standards that weren't my own and when I got sick, the determination I felt to make up for what I lacked was stronger than ever. I was beating myself up for not being "normal" and not having the family everybody wanted me to have with beautiful children and a Roth IRA. I was angry at myself and everyone around me for why I was broken and alone. I wanted someone real, someone willing to love me for my shattered mind and heart. I needed someone to be patient with me the way my dad never was or tell me I was beautiful without commenting on my outward appearance like my mother always did. Someone to take the time to teach me so I could learn without feeling rushed. I hated that my addiction convinced me that I needed someone to do all of these things so I could be made whole.

When I witnessed my ex helping my other ex move out of my house, I was sparked with curiosity about how he was doing and why Leo had called him to help. I guess it was normal for my ex-lovers to come together as friends; how could they not with how small the town was? I did what any normal person would do and stalked his Instagram to see what he was up to. It's not like I could have offered him a coffee or anything since he was driving my ex-husband away in his car. I was baffled to see him living life sober since the last I heard from him he was doing heroin and stealing gold teeth from his patients since he worked as a mortician at a local funeral home. I scrolled through his pictures and saw a mix between his graffiti work and NA outings with friends. I had never heard of NA (Narcotics Anonymous) before and thought that it must really work if my ex got clean and sober. I didn't think anything of it until I randomly got a DM from him asking how I was doing and how he was sorry for showing up at my place unannounced. I was surprised to have gotten a message from and a tad skeptical that Instagram knows how to let people know that you were just peeping their profiles, when I replied with a question of "What is NA?"

Yes, alcohol was good while it lasted, but I had already kicked the drinking. Marijuana was yummy when I needed it, but it was no longer a preferred method to numb the pain, and I only liked cocaine if I was drinking, so take away the drinking and the blow naturally cancels itself out. Sex, however…sex was something I wasn't desperate enough to give up even though I had stooped to the lowest point of who I was having sex with. I wasn't ready to identify as a sex addict even though I knew I was addicted to people—addicted to having sex with those people. As Brad Pitt says in *Fight Club* "self-improvement is masturbation, but self-destruction…." he never finishes his sentence but I believe self-destruction is where you really learn about yourself and I was learning so much much about myself while wrapped up in the sheets.

I showed up to my first meeting with a pious attitude and thought that I was nothing like these heavy drug users. Some of them ended up on the streets and some had been convicted felons. I thought that just because I sat pretty in a two-story house I was better off than they were. I chose a chair furthest from the door to sit in so I could get an unobstructed view of the room just in case I saw anyone I needed to hide from. I wasn't sure I belonged there for any other purpose than to shop for my next piece of ass when I saw a few familiar faces walk through the door. Around a circled table sat a group of different people including some girls I knew from high school, my ex-lover, and my little league soccer coach. Quite the crowd, I thought, when I saw a new face walk through the door. I wasn't aware that my intention for showing up would slowly change into showing up for myself, but before that took place, I had to ruin my life just one more time.

Chapter 11

#NAthroughosmosis#addictionkills

The rooms of NA were helping me gain some introspection as to why I was doing what I was doing, and one of the things I learned was that I had gone from cheering for the underdog to hating people who were always happy and routing for the underdog. I constantly flip-flopped and couldn't decide whether I wanted to play the bully or the victim. Perhaps it was because I secretly wanted someone to cheer me on but never appropriately felt it from those closest to me. I felt the support from strangers at my church when I went, but there is nothing like having your loved ones feed you your encouragement. I despised people who wanted nothing more than to be positive all the time and breeze through negative emotions as if they didn't exist; those were the people I gave the most shit to. I loved being the one to remind them that life isn't all sunshine and rainbows, but the burden of pain that never goes away. My ignorance was bliss, and for that, my self-destruction was ignored for fear of having to take ownership of it. No one seemed to want to claim the fires they started and even with a program like NA, it was hard to raise my hand and tell the truth. But that's exactly what I did when I saw others do it. I always had this desire for others to acknowledge their bad so I didn't have to acknowledge mine alone, and I finally felt safe enough to share my own experiences.

I kept showing up to meetings, and each time I left the fluorescent-lit room, I learned something I didn't know about myself and the world around me. Narcotics Anonymous is a 12-step program that follows principles and structure to help an addict live life clean. They say cleanliness is close to Godliness and having a higher power in your corner is one of the vital steps in beating your addiction. Getting ahead of it like you're in a race and all your temptations are trying to tie you for first place. Some prayers were recited at the meetings, something I was familiar with, and a code of honor to keep to ensure that I was in a safe space. I hadn't been going to Sage Church, so this was exactly what I needed. I would hear stories from other addicts that helped me take mental notes about how I was more like everyone in the room than not. It was during one of the meetings that his green eyes began to burn through my skin, distracting me from the message. He was my type and my favorite kind of distraction.

I met Rupert when I walked outside after a meeting one night while smoking a cigarette with all the other NA-goers. I wasn't really a smoker, but when in Rome. The 6 '2, green-eyed distraction was now on my radar and just like the rest, he was easy on the eyes and came with boatloads of trauma. You are what you attract, they say. You are what you eat, they say. I hate how "they" are right. Never mind that I had just gone through some serious trauma with sex being at the center of it; it was second nature for me to move on and get creative with it. I wasn't about to pass up Rupert just because I was learning about the meaning of addiction. If anything, he was my way into obtaining sobriety further. Why couldn't I just go after a nice guy that wasn't an addict? Why couldn't I just have stayed single?! Why?! Why?! Why?!

I was afraid to go after anyone who wasn't like me - anyone who wasn't an addict. A clean-cut man with moral values and a level head didn't seem within my reach, or it just meant that I would have a boring life of consistency and discipline. I wasn't willing to put myself out there when I knew I couldn't measure up to a man who would be my rock. Settling into a relationship with someone who could aid me with becoming a person of substance while simultaneously accepting my flaws didn't sound anything short of science fiction. So I settled for Rupert. Rupert walked over to me as I was mingling with some new friends and offered a sly remark about my beauty. It was your typical cat-and-mouse chase that ended with our phone numbers entered into each other's phones.

Over the next couple of days, Rupert and I texted back and forth, getting to know each other. That is when I learned he was from a Mormon family and had three kids from two different women. I quickly saw some similarities that he shared with my father, but I honestly wasn't worried about him having kids since they weren't around much since Rupert lost custody of them after he was charged with a lengthy list of crimes. Could I really have expected anything less from a hypersexual, meth addict that had just been released from jail? It was nice to learn about someone else's story other than my own calamitous story. I was truly fascinated by Rupert's testimony and he was just getting started.

Rupert had been on house arrest and lived in a very sketchy apartment complex that also functioned as a hotel. The guy was horrible on paper but I had compassion for his trials. I did my best to see the good inside each lover of mine after they saw the inside of me, between my thighs. That was how it was with my encounters. If I wanted to know you on a deeper level, I had to let go deep inside of me for you to open up. And after that, you'd dish your idiosyncrasies and show me who you are. Something like, "I'll show you mine if you show me yours." I wanted Rupert's heart and was feeling excited to have someone new in my life after Leo, but before I won him over, I had to prance around to hype up the chase. Rupert had no idea what he was in for with me punishing him or stepping all over his heart if he didn't bow down to my every need. All he thought we were doing was going on our first date.

The noise of the restaurant gave us some privacy so Rupert and I could share our drama over some beans and rice. We were sitting from each other when he first mentioned that he had a curfew and had to be home by 8 PM, which explained why he chose a restaurant across the street from his apartment. Then he shared with me some, but not all, the details about his criminal charges when my phone rang and interrupted him. I ignored the call so he could continue, but at that point he deflected and turned the attention over to me. I was still holding my phone when I received a text from my mom about my brother being arrested. My initial reaction was to get upset, but then I realized how overplayed this was. Jax and I hadn't been on speaking terms ever since he set his car on fire in my driveway. What did he do this time? With how many times Jax had been in trouble, I was losing sight of each offense. I would always tell people Jax was my twin; that we were one and the same, except he got caught all the time.

I looked up from my phone and Rupert caught my facial expression, quickly shifting his mood to mirror mine. I took less than a second to decide if I should milk this situation to lure Rupert in deeper. I used to think that any opportunity for a guy to see my eyes change colors with glistening tears rolling down my face would surely pull them closer to me. I let a single crocodile tear roll off my cheek and acted stunned before telling Rupert about Jax going to jail. Rupert hugged me and asked if I wanted to go to his place to smoke a cig and talk about it. Before I answered, a flash went through my mind, only to land on the question "Was I going to sleep with him tonight?" My internal dialog answered yes, so I told Rupert that I was game to go to his place to talk. I started to shift my demeanor into a woman with a secret as I approached his door and reminded myself that I really did have something to tell him that I thought would determine whether or not he would want to sleep with me.

I was sitting on Rupert's bed, since his place was basically one giant bedroom and there was no furniture to sit on, when I thought about revealing my shaved head to him. I began flirting with him while twirling my fake hair, thinking to myself that I was finally going to be rejected because my looks were not up to code. Long hair has been the staple to a man's arousal since the beginning of time. Would I turn him off if I told him the truth? This was the first time I had ever feared sexual rejection from a man.

"Promise you won't lie to me and you'll tell me what you think about what I'm about to show you?"

"Yes, I promise. You have me so intrigued! I have no clue what you are about to say."

"It's not what I'm going to say, it's what I'm going to show you!"

"Show me?"

"Close your eyes."

"Now I'm scared! Haha!"

As he covered his face with a pillow, I took off my wig and gave him the go-ahead to look. He took one look at me as I hung my head low, refusing to make eye contact with him because I felt shame over my hairstyle choice. The long hair I used as my security blanket was gone and I felt that my looks had been compromised. He asked if he could touch my head after he smiled at me, so I let him. Rupert began telling me I really created such suspense for the base to drop in a way he wasn't expecting. He liked it. After a sigh of relief and some discussion about my decision to shave my head, I felt free to release more of my secrets. That night was a night of freedom I hadn't ever experienced before. I had never been so forthcoming with my truth even though I was manipulating how I told that truth. I wasn't ready for organic truth. I learned in NA that there is a difference between bragging and admitting I was mixing the two for a justifiable reason. I wanted to disguise my feelings with the defense of bragging about my truths instead of admitting my decision to hurt myself or Rupert.

After I let Rupert pet my head, I knew it was time to test the waters and push the boundaries to see if this guy would still like me after all was said and done. I hadn't known I was dealing with a fellow sex addict and he would do just about anything to get his fix too. I told Rupert about one more thing I thought would disturb him and that was that I had tattooed my ex-husband's name over my pelvis. Full-on vagina ink claiming Leo's territory. I had let Leo tattoo his name on me as a gesture of good faith after we got engaged; the shit I did to convince others of my loyalty was outstanding, given I had no real intention of staying within bounds.

Rupert snarked at me and asked, "Can I see it?" As you can

imagine, I said yes and allowed my inner carnivorous animal to come out and play for the rest of the night. The type of sex we had was the very type of sex that unleashed my addiction further. For the next week, I had been hooked, lined, and sinking slowly with Rupert. We were inseparable after we slept with each other and started to show up to meetings together. We were talking around the clock about anything and everything, and to me, Rupert was the cat's meow. I thought Rupert was good for me with the way he challenged my verbiage and taught me more about recovery. I loved that about him. He had been in the program for a year before I showed up and he always made it a point to prioritize the principles of recovery in his life.

One afternoon I was hanging out with a girlfriend when I got a call from Leo. It had only been three weeks since we had broken up, and I was doing everything to avoid him. I didn't know it was him since he changed his number after I commandeered the car, but I knew it was him once I heard his voice raging on the other side.

"How could you M.K.?"

"What the fuck are you talking about?"

"How could you let that creep fuck you?"

"Who I'm fucking is my business and what do you care? It's over."

"You know the guy is a child molester, right?"

"What?!"

Leo began sharing with me how a friend of his at NA told him about Rupert's charges. Rupert never got to that part during our date, if he was going to tell me at all, so I got the privilege of hearing it from my ex-husband.

"Simon told me that Rupert was in jail for molesting some teenage girl and is a registered sex offender!"

"Was Simon also the one to tell you we've been seeing each other?"

"M.K. it doesn't matter how I found out. Just Google the guy. You'll get all your facts and know I'm not just saying this to mess with you."

"If this is your attempt at getting back with me, you really need some new material."

"M.K. I'm serious. I may hate you right now but I don't want anything bad to happen to you."

"Fine. I'll look him up."

So I did. I sat on my friend's bed and pulled up *Rupert Macabee* on my phone in the Google search box and a list of headlines appeared below his name that explained each charge that Rupert had, including the words **Registered Sex Offender** in red letters. I clicked on the link which took me to a site containing his mugshot (which was unflattering) and information about all known sex offenders in my area. Leo was right. I was appalled, disgusted, and so pissed off that he didn't tell me since he had plenty of opportunities to come clean. I wasn't sure if I should call him to reprimand him or wait for him to get off of work to seize a window for punishment. I told myself I could go by his work and make a scene, but I knew that if I did that, I would risk my image of being the sweet M.K. who gets free carwashes since everyone at the carwash liked me. I asked my girlfriend what I should do and she told me that I should just call him right then and there. So I did.

"Hey, pretty lady!"

"Is it true?"

"I'm not following."

"You know exactly what I'm talking about."

"I think we should talk about this in person."

"How dare you not tell me, you sick piece of shit!"

"M.K. I can explain…."

"What's there to explain? I read all about it online!"

"Do you want to hear my side or not?"

"I'll be at your place at eight."

I hung up the phone and pulled myself together to prepare for our meeting. Rupert—the NA boy who works as a manager at a carwash that I can't help but be attracted to. Deep down, I thought he was a total loser, something of a diamond in the rough with how sexy he was, but I was about to learn that Rupert and I weren't so different and his charges were not going to stop me from going back for more.

I showed up at his house that evening and we did our normal ritual of sitting across from each other in his tiny room, lighting our cigarettes. American Spirits to be exact, and if you have ever smoked one from a turquoise box, then you know how winded I felt after taking a long, steady drag. I wasn't sure if I should have been upset or started talking like I was upset since it was hard to regain my ground when I was around Rupert. I let my cigarette dangle from between my fingers before letting out a "SO??..." and he began to ramble on about how sorry he was. He told me how he was waiting for the right moment to share the heinous facts about himself and how hurt he was that I found out the way I did. I countered his apology by saying he had plenty of chances to tell me, but I knew that I wasn't as offended as I was leading on. I really liked Rupert but he didn't know that. I know that I was guilty of indulging in his panic but that was just like me: watching the worm squirm before throwing it in my mouth. After he finished sharing his very detailed story of feeling up a teenager, I couldn't help but be compelled by his candor. By no means was I dismissive of what he had done, but there was a new feeling I was experiencing for Rupert and the sorrow I felt in his voice. I had never been that sorry for an offense I'd committed like he was and it left me deeply touched - and that much more attracted to him.

Rupert was a perfect combination of the men I had loved before and the fact that he had been sexually involved with men, like all the rest, made me confident our traumas would get along. It was more obvious to me that I had a type for men who were grimy, vulgar, and wicked handsome with some intellect. But most importantly, they were obsessed with me. No different than me doing everything to take back control from what I had lost when I was a little girl, the men I was dating were doing the same. We all had a common bond, and that was sexual trauma. No wonder Rupert and I loved sharing our sex addiction; we weren't ready to do anything about it and it made for some memorable times until I made the first move to push him away. It was always self-sabotage to sabotage my relationships and that came in the form of a chiseled physique on top of me that wasn't Rupert.

Rupert had been planning on seeing his kids for the first time since he was released from jail and things were getting serious when the idea of introducing me to his children was on the table. I had mixed feelings about it and so did he, but since Rupert and I were not on the same page when it came to our future and family together, tensions were rising. I was blunt with him about wanting to try for another child on our second date but Rupert was done having kids, so I just shrugged it off like he wasn't my forever person yet, I kept telling myself I wanted him to be. I noticed Rupert had mixed emotions about introducing his children to me and was extremely shut down one night, to the point of causing a fight. He refused to talk to me about what was going on with him and I took that as a slap to the face. Why wasn't he opening up to me? I couldn't seem to get a reaction out of him so I took the rejection as a reason to place a wedge between us. I stormed out of his musty apartment and walked to my car only to pull out my phone and open up my Tinder app. I hadn't used it since Leo and I broke up, so I had to patiently wait for it to redownload, giving me plenty of time to rethink my decision. Nothing made me more determined than a man rejecting me. My hurt feelings made me want to hurt his feelings back.

I drove away while the app downloaded, and once I got to my place I was on the swipe til I got it right, if you know what I mean. I knew I had a way of indirectly teaching others but when a frat boy showed up to my place, I thought I was going to be coaching him more than I was playing with him. Mr. 18-year-old came inside and had me blown away by his confidence. I thought I was just going to act out and perform my number to rock this guy's world with my pornographic tendencies, but instead I was the one who got her world rocked.

It was the moment that my one-night stand squared up to me and said, "Look at you, you just want to be loved, don't you?" that I had felt truly embarrassed for how desperate I was; obvious enough for him to notice. It wasn't enough that he made me orgasm without me having to filter myself, which never happens with one-hitter-quitters, but I was also able to just be myself for the first time ever. My desperate self. I let every truth I had burried down within me come out in the form of vulnerable sex and desperation. Being desperate really is the hardest state that I've ever been in, and it wasn't easy but it made being a trauma victim feel like I could move on easily. The night terrors, memories, and visions can always be replaced, but being desperate for love, healthy and appropriate love, felt irreplacable. Wanting love had me swinging wild to do anything I could to get my hands on it. I wish I would have known the horror my desperation was about to cause me because it would go down in history as the worst thing I've ever felt.

I woke up the next day and headed to work at a studio/spa where I taught a belly dancing class (which was good for me since I was shining a light on Type 1 diabetes by wearing my medical device on my belly for all to see). After my class, I texted Rupert, asking him if we were doing our usual hang session after we both got off work, and got no response. I wanted to sting him by telling him what I did, but I also started to let my conscious get the best of me and began to regret what I had done. What was happening to me? Do I tell him what happened with false modesty or do I just keep it to myself? I had a burning desire to tell him what I was suffering from but was afraid he would leave me. I waited all day for his response until he finally invited me over for dinner.

Rupert was silent after I came clean to him about my night with the college boy. I could tell the gears were turning in his mind, but still, he said nothing. The whole reason I felt like I should cheat on him was a massive discovery for me and I wanted to share that with him. More silence. I was triggered by his silence and his shutting down was such a jab to the stomach that I felt he was perpetuating the damage. Anger has many faces and being silent is one of them. Here we were again. He thanked me for telling him the truth before we got into a deep conversation about our sex addictions. It's not like he didn't know from my past indiscretions which, in my opinion, I laid out like a perfectly trimmed warning sign. That's so like me, to gaslight my lover. I thought he knew I was unfit for monogamy but I tried my best to let him know that my heart longed for him and the only way he could interpret that was to take my clothes off. I noticed he was being more aggressive than usual, and when I started to feel more pain than pleasure, I knew something was wrong.

I looked up at Rupert with my eyes squinted from the pain I felt, which didn't seem to phase him. It was as if he wanted to see my face in pain, my body in pain, and he knew that his thrusting was doing the trick. It was when he tossed me like a rag doll onto my belly that I felt the shift in our sex dynamic. He was revenge fucking me. Rupert told me we were going to do anal and spread my legs apart as I dug my head into his comforter. He was gentle in the beginning, but then he got sharper with each undulation. I remember thinking to myself that I deserved his aggression because of what I did to him and allowing him to do this to me was a way to get back in his good graces. What a warped way to look at the person I'd been saying "I love you" to.

After he was done, I went right back to feeling disassociated as I had always felt after sex. I thought I was making headway in coming back to my real feelings in my very real body and then this happened. I didn't know what to do other than to make a joke to lighten the mood since using humor to mask how I was really feeling was what I did best. Rupert told me he wanted to be alone for the rest of the night, so I left. I wanted so badly to tell him how I was really feeling but I never bared my true self. Instead, my true self went home and cried about what he had done. I felt so sad that I had stooped so low but it didn't warrant him violating me. There was no respect or comfort and I should have said something. I was starting to wake up to my power of saying "NO" and I couldn't fall back into walking around in a slumber if I was going to turn my life around.

I had been sober from alcohol and drugs and had been learning how to live in my new, sick body a little more every day, why couldn't I start to address my sex addiction?! It was time to say "NO" more than I was saying "YES" to men. Omitting what had happened with Rupert was not an option, and I was ready to address what went down. I called a friend of mine to help counsel me into finding healing and remembered that I didn't have to face this alone. I was done living the lie that sex was something dismal and life-ruining, that it was meant to be beautiful and cherished. If I wanted any shot of having something healthy for myself and my sex life, I needed to stand up for ME and keep my self-love intact. I lost sight of all the work I had slowly been putting in towards redefining who I was. I thought I was nothing more than a mean girl. A gossip. Someone who says too much and comes off too strong. I never acted professionally, and I was always looking to set people up for a trap. I was someone who blamed others all the time and couldn't stay away from sex.

If someone asked me what I saw when I looked in the mirror, I would say that I saw caramel-colored eyes and grapefruit-pink lips. But when I looked deeper, I saw pain and endurance; a beautiful child of God with such fight in her soul, always pressing on to see the beauty in everything. I saw trauma trying to cloud out all the light. Insecure and afraid, I saw a woman who had moments of despair and felt out of place. A child acting out to be heard and waiting to be told things were going to be OK. Once I was OK, I saw a woman changing and evolving. A misunderstood, God-given magic only He could help me learn to use. A believer stared back at me in the mirror, and when I looked upon that girl from day to day, I saw how she appeared different by the moment. I was a loose cannon one minute and super composed the next. The symptoms of a girl turning into a woman, growing up in such harsh conditions, can find rest in all that is seen outside of the mirror. I finally saw God and his light shine through my soul when I looked in the mirror the night I went to talk to Rupert. I wasn't consumed with my flawed skin or the value my face held. For the first time in my life, I accepted the woman I saw reflecting back at me. I decided to be brave and tell Rupert my truth.

His apology was empty and he reacted with disregard for my feelings. Perhaps he felt the same way I did when I apologized to him. Half-fake but half-true. I was hoping we could put all of this behind us and be stronger for it but when I saw his lack of remorse, his entitlement for having his way with me, I knew it was time to let him go. My friends wanted me to ditch him and my family had wanted me to ditch him even more once it was out that the chief's daughter was dating a registered sex offender. Rupert had me though. I was addicted. His humor, warm chiseled body, the chainsmoking, and the acrobatic love making were just too good to pass up. It was all of it. I did not want to let go, which is why I continued to stay with him even after his reaction. My fear of being alone and giving up my drug had me feeling the exact same symptoms as when I got diagnosed with T1D. Heart palpitations and cold sweat showed kicking my love and sex addiction was just as scary to me as wondering if I was going to accidentally OD on my insulin injection. If I wanted to see the benefits of a life uncompromised with my own self-worth and respect, then I needed to draw some boundaries. It was always a compromise, a trade-off in my mind, for why I deserved the worst of someone, and setting boundaries for myself was unheard of.

It had been a week after our incident that something fascinating happened to me. Rupert and I were complacent in our relationship and I had already begun to disconnect from him when I met Micah. Rupert and I were talking about my past run-ins with famous people, and I had been explaining to him that it wasn't that hard to meet someone famous if he wanted to. I was going on and on about the laws of attraction, and later that day, I was working at the studio when in walked this 5 '10, brown-eyed, man with a jawline that screamed 'model'. At first glance, he was not my type but I couldn't let his gentle "Do you know where the spa is?" be ignored. When I made eye contact with him I politely told him to follow me towards the spa. As I walked in front of him, I felt the scan he gave me down my exposed spine, and when we approached the spa, I opened the door for him to walk through. He seemed very smitten by me from the smile he shot at me before thanking me for helping him. I had walked away knowing he was going to be thinking about me while he got his massage. I, however, was not going to give him a second thought and rushed off back to the studio for class.

I had just finished class when Micah met me at the front desk of the studio. I had been checking emails when I saw a hand land on the counter with a sliver of paper peeking out from under it. I looked away from my screen to check what was on the paper, and I saw a phone number with a name written down. So, I looked up and saw the pretty boy smiling at me, asking me if I would like to get tea sometime, to give him a call, as he slid the paper towards me.

I picked it up and said "OK, Micah," and watched him walk away. The second he was out of hearing range all of my coworkers rushed over to me, completely in awe of what they had just witnessed.

"Do you know who that was?!"

"No."

"That was Micah Vino! The actor, duh!"
"Micah who?"

"The guy from *Vampire Diaries.*"

My coworkers flocked around me to take over my computer and pulled up *Micah Vino* in the search engine with disbelief that I didn't know who he was. I was already skeptical about Googling guys' names but what was the worst that could happen? I find out he's a serial killer? I watched all the women scroll through the info that was attached to his name and was surprised to see how popular Micah was—and how expensive. Clearly, I wasn't a fangirl of his, but perhaps one in the making. I'd give him a text to know more about him, but my heart and body were still yearning for Rupert. I had been going to therapy for a few sessions after my epiphany with my identity crisis when I told my therapist about Micah. It amazes me that I had been going to therapy on and off since I was 13 and was still excited to showcase my narcissistic talents. I wasn't ready to be rewired but I loved storytelling, and I was over the moon to tell Dr. "What's Her Face" about my run-in with Micah in hopes she could help me decipher my next course of action.

Let's face it: can you really help someone who doesn't want to be helped? I told her I wanted to tell Rupert about the encounter, to brag of course, but then turn around and rip Micah's number up as a grandiose gesture of my loyalty and love. It should've been just enough theater to assure him that he was the only guy for me. As I sat in my chair with the ugliest decorative pillow, my therapist nodded in amusement and told me to trust myself to make the right decision. The right decision was to save Micah's number in my phone before I went to Rupert's place that night, and did exactly what I had intended to do. Rupert was stunned, yet happy I was so convinced about wanting to play house with some more, without any distractions. I waited a couple of days before reaching out to Micah and he was quick to suggest a meetup time and place, so I wasted no time preparing myself.

Micah had been in town filming a show on the WB and was looking for some authentic, Fanta Se while he was there. Who better to give him a personal tour than me? Micah pulled up in his fully loaded Rubicon as I wrestled my pups at a park. I was wearing a comfy dress that stretched over my curvy body and my favorite cut-off hoodie.

When he hopped out of his Jeep and started to walk over to where I was, I thought I would meet him halfway so he could see the sun hitting my face just right. The sweat glistened on my face and chest as we met in the middle of a grassy field. There was no awkward lean-in for a hug, just heavy eye contact. After greeting each other, Micah asked if I wanted to go for a ride, so I walked my dogs back home and headed out with who I thought was the perfect stranger.

The sun was setting and we cruised to some of my favorite spots around town. I was proud to show him my stomping grounds whilst sharing a sunset together, but it was when I took him to our last stop at the top of High Road that I began to play fortune teller and knew Micah was going to want to see me again. We drove up a street that led to some bougie homes and a dead end that overlooked the city lights. There was a wall that divided the housing from the desert that we hoodlums used to climb back in the day to sit and stare at the lights as we puffed our joints. High Road was called High Road for a reason, and I wanted Micah and I to share our first date with some realness. "Real" usually gets real, so once I exposed my vulnerable side to Micah, I hoped he would do the same. We jumped up on the wall to see each beaming light stare back at us with the backdrop of mountains forming a bowl that looked as if we were trapped in it. We laughed and shared some common beliefs as we agreed that being Mexican-Americans whose fathers were in law enforcement wasn't easy. I felt like I had finally started to attract someone who could bring out the better version of me. The side of me that wasn't constantly in survival mode with vindictive behavior on repeat. It felt good to be subtle and not so aggressive on a first date.

After my night with Micah, I was sure that I wanted to see him again. If I didn't sleep with him or kiss him, could I still go on dates with him and it NOT be considered cheating? It was cheating with how intentional I was with my emotions around Micah and I knew that both him and Rupert wouldn't like knowing about each other, so I was just going to keep it to myself. I didn't care about Micah being an actor; he strummed my strings that Rupert failed to touch. I looked at it as if I were balancing both men in my life and I wanted them both. Rupert was my "sure thing" and Micah was my mystery. This looked like Leo and Ara in the making all over again, and if I didn't play it smart, my outcome would surely be a disaster. Is there ever a smart way to be insane? How long would it last this time? I'd been there many times before and it always ended the same. But spoken like a true addict, I was going to do it anyway. I had been steadily going to therapy and attending my NA meetings every week, but having a sponsor to hold me accountable for the decisions I was making was what was missing. I needed help before I hurt myself again.

I left work early one day and went to see Rupert at work and to get my car washed when I noticed a lifted Rubicon in front of me. My blood left my face as I stood outside my car, emptying my trash, when Micah stepped down from his Jeep and looked in my direction. I immediately wanted to turn around but the traffic jam suggested otherwise. I was stuck in line and my only option was to go with it. My many personalities and I were scrambling to come up with a solution when I saw Rupert exit the side door where his office was located and head towards me. Rupert had a smile on his face as he strutted my way and I did my best to try not to notice him. I appeared busy, throwing away important paperwork and car items I had every intention of keeping when Rupert was gaining in on me. I felt a light touch on my shoulder and a "Hey babe," from none other than Micah. Rupert had almost made it to my car when I turned around to face Micah, giving

Rupert my 'once sec' finger, signaling I'd be with him in a moment. Rupert gave me the most confused look and walked away to help a customer.

Micah let go of me and scanned me up and down to compliment my outfit when I thanked him with a hug. I wonder if he noticed the horror in my eyes and the suffocating panic I was experiencing! I let out a faint "Thank you" and told him I had to run inside real quick, doing my best to pace myself walking through the lot. Once I got inside, I beelined to the bathroom to sit and hyperventilate for a second. What was I going to do? The bathroom started closing in on me as I thought about the last time this happened to me. I felt like God gave me an opportunity to come clean with those two when they had just missed each other the time before this. Did I take the hint? No, not at all. So there I was. I took a deep breath and rehearsed my lines before finding Rupert to explain myself. I walked out into the lobby, which was made up of 90% window, only to see the two boys talking to each other side by side.

I peeked through a window, attempting to read their body language, and with a dry mouth all I thought about was how I felt like I was a little girl again, about to get in trouble with my dad. Funny how these issues come full circle. Rupert stood next to Micah, towering over him with his 6 '2 stance and arms crossed while Micah stood adjacent to Rupert, using his hands as he spoke. It seemed like Rupert had a frown on his face but there was no way to tell for sure with how often his body was shifting out of view. I watched the conversation come to an end as Micah got into his Jeep and drove away (in a heated manner, judging by the sound of his screeching tires). I used that as my cue to step outside and meet Rupert. He knew a saucy story was coming his way as I did my best to wipe off the cowardly residue on my clothes.

You would think that I figured out that my cheating and manipulation weren't going to help the panic attacks or tame my cortisol spikes by living in a constant state of fear of getting caught, but no. Nothing stopped me. Micah called me as soon as I walked back to my car and fed me a mouthful. I didn't need any more boy drama, so it was time to come clean. I was going to dump Rupert and focus on getting my core beliefs in line. It was time to settle down, and the next guy I got involved with, I told myself, would be my last.

Chapter 12

#Kstandsforindispenable#potassium

There are a few people in your life, if you're lucky, that will impact you and the way you live in a healthy and positive way. It's the way they show up for you, the lessons they teach you, and the lengths they are willing to go through that show their brand of love, making you feel blessed to have them in your life. I had felt that way about every person I chose to love and be intimate with in the beginning and in the end - never in the middle. The middle always made me feel like I was trapped in the thick of the game where all pieces on the board were aligned for attack, exposed for the checkmate. When each of these relationships/encounters came to an end, I didn't believe I could walk away with a lesson that would eventually lead to my recovery until now. If it weren't for the tragic love stories or the heartache that brought me to my knees, I wouldn't have an attitude of gratefulness for walking away with my life. Every single person that came into my life brought both beauty and travesty to teach me this one lesson: I can love myself without being loved by many.

Rupert was one of those men who taught me how to stay close to God by having alone time with Him and I thanked him for that before we went our separate ways. I found a sponsor through NA, which is someone who has had a couple of years or more under their belt of clean time, that helps you follow your stepwork through the program. My sponsor came in the form of a female who advised me to replace the word drug or alcohol in the NA text with the word SEX. It made sense for my case since I was living life as well as I could by being an active sex addict. It didn't matter that I had four years of sobriety from drugs and booze when the real culprit was between my legs. It wasn't enough to finally seek out therapy from a therapist who knew I couldn't bullshit my way through my sessions (since she had a rule about my clean time before seeing me). I was told that the first year of sobriety was the year I would come back into my body and realize what the fuck was going on - my wake-up phase, if you will. The second year was the year of depicting what was what and identifying what I knew to be true. What the truth is by common standards. The third year is when I would pull it together to accomplish goals and keep a steady pace, living life on life's terms without blaming the world for my problems. Thus came my fourth year of really wanting to put in the work and learning how to break free from my sex addiction after finally admitting that it was a serious problem of mine.

I learned so much about myself through my step work and through my therapy sessions that I began to feel overloaded with the truths about my life. It felt like a relapse was one more harsh truth about myself away from happening and I was reminded of why I started drinking and drugging to begin with. I was journaling about why I was doing what I was doing and all the deep-seated trauma that set me up for the nasty path I took. It was harsh, and I was ready to go in the opposite direction and transition to a healthy way of thinking so that I could fight off the temptation of using people as an escape. I was constantly escaping from one lover to the next. I had to chase my recovery like I chased my men if I was going to quit my *escape* act. Micah had seen my internal battle with myself and labeled me a hot mess after he circled around and found his way back to me. There was always the gravitational pull regardless of how messy I was. He caught on and no matter how hard I tried to salvage my friendship with him, he suggested I read *The Untethered Soul* by Michael Singer and bid me farewell. Rejection had become a teacher for me, and I found myself humbled after Micah and I went our separate ways. I hadn't slept with Micah, and that was a first for me. It's not that he didn't want to nor that I didn't want to, it was my emotional episodes that prevented anything from happening. I was falling apart more often than not, and I felt like my growing pains were never going to end. I hadn't known that I was undergoing the greatest transformation by putting in the work to better my spiritual mind and body. I was asking myself questions like, "Why am I so unfulfilled in relationships?" and "Why am I giving away what is so precious to me, so freely?"

My reality was that I wasn't making my partners work for me or my vagina. I was barely working towards myself, so wearing my heart on my sleeve was causing my sleeves to get shorter and shorter. I wondered why the men I chose never really kept up with me and my interests or why they just stopped picking my brain altogether. It was as if I was obsolete after they received their primal needs. The honeymoon phase always seemed to die out as quickly as it started, and I was beginning to think that I wasn't interesting enough. All the self-confidence I had was overshadowed by my insecurities, and after Rupert cheated on me, I knew that our relationship was surely going to come to an end. The saying "once a cheater, always a cheater" couldn't have been more up to code with how the rest of our relationship played out.

Micah stepped away from me after all the drama, which I understood, being that he was in the limelight and the only drama he wanted was scripted on paper and filmed for cash. Rupert had attempted to hook up with Carla to get back at me for causing drama, and now I was looking for a way to feel needed since the people I chose to grow closest to didn't want me close any longer. They did, but they didn't, if you know what I mean. I had to break up with Rupert, which left me homeless since we had been living together. That meant I had to run to Carla, who housed me until I met a slew of new people to help carry me through my turbulent time. It was chaos! There was William and Raven and a no-namer along the way, and there was love and hate and attempts to stay in church when I finally crash-landed back where I took off from— Rupert's.

When is enough, enough? Rupert was madly in love with me and I loved him too, but in the worst way. The only way I felt I could leave him alone for good was to find my soulmate, my twin flame, the guy who made other men want to be more like him. The sweet man who wouldn't dare raise his voice at me or lay a hand on me. The gentleman who saw me for me, knew when to be available for me, and not judge me for wanting my needs met. I wanted a sober man who would make love to me and not just treat my body as if it were a pitstop for his carnal needs, instead a temple to pray in and grow closer to love in. I didn't think I deserved that kind of man after all I had been through, and as much as I was learning about my addiction, I was succumbing to it just to get by. Getting back together with Rupert was my final attempt to keep a stable roof over my head and a body to cuddle for reassurance. My need for skin-on-skin attention was past the point of needing it; I was craving it.

I first saw Kaden at a meeting where he sat across from me at the last supper table, as I liked to refer to it, with his big blue eyes staring at me. They were the bluest eyes I had ever seen, and I'd seen four different bodies of water. Still, nothing could explain those eyes. I saw Rupert on a couch right behind Kaden and noticed Rupert had me in his line of view to peek at me. Once I locked eyes with Kaden, nothing else mattered. I watched Kaden watching me as I ate some of my emergency, low-blood sugar candy and how his eyes followed every move I made. I smiled at Kaden right as Rupert looked over at me, thinking the smile was intended for him. Surely, Rupert would have noticed that my eyes weren't on him but in my peripherals. Kaden smiled back at me and no matter how hard I tried, I could not detach myself from Kaden's ocean blue eyes. Something told me that those waves would soon take me under, and I would drown.

The thing about finding a lover in NA, or in a small town in general, is that 8/10 times people double-dipped. It was hard to meet someone who hadn't been with someone you had already been with. That alone is a brain tongue twister. Kaden had been dating a fellow NA goer named Lacy, and I respected that enough to stay away from doing what I normally would do when I wanted to capture a man. Even though I had been with Rupert, I knew that Kaden was going to be the last man I'd ever be with. The cosmos were aligned and Kaden was going to be mine. That's how perfect I knew this guy was at first sight. It was undeniable when our eyes met or we hugged that an inferno of desire would heat up the room. Everyone knew it. Everyone hated it. Especially Rupert and Lacy. I had never been patient long enough to let the forces of nature split two people up before I went in for the kill. It was always: I see, I zone in, I conquer. This time, I was going to be patient and let Kaden and Lacy break up by Lacy proving how unfit she was for him. I humbly sat on the sidelines and waited, something I had never done before.

Kaden had a friend named Britani who I totally had a crush on and loved being around. I knew I couldn't pursue Britani since I broke away from being bisexual and devoted my spiritual body to being strictly man and woman through my Christian faith, but that didn't mean I denied the psychology of the human mind. If I were alive when Jesus was I'd ask Him if He had to choose one, which would He choose? Psychology or religion? I'd bet He would answer psychology given He understood the complexities of the mind and how beautifully made we are as children of God. He knew were fallen with our warped minds in need of a savior. He knew religion just made everyone a hypocrite, so giving up my desire for women was all in good faith, not to mention how overwhelming loving both men and women in relationships had proven to be for me. Britani was not going to be my next quest but my new best friend. It didn't hurt that she was also Kaden's best friend. I knew I wanted to play fair but I was still a sex addict at the end of the day.

Being a sex and love addict is like harvesting a plant. First, a seed of desire is planted, then the growth exploration, and finally you reap the benefit of whatever forbidden fruit you planted. This season's crops were tainted and I was about to find out why. After befriending Britani, she soon became someone I genuinely cared about after a few months of spending time with her. She would visit me 45 minutes away from where she lived and tell me secrets that I cradled with care, something I wasn't known for. But Britani was special to me. It was rare for me to have such a sincere relationship with a female considering that all the females in my life had betrayed me before I got a chance to turn the tables on them. I was doing my part to make sure to mind my pints and quarts with this friendship. Brit was reviving my belief in what it meant to have a friend and BE a friend.

One of the unique things about Britani was that she was soon to become a he—Carter. Brit was making moves to transition and became my first transgender friend, going through a series of medical appointments that overwhelmed her to no end. I had a chance to show up and be a supportive friend when Brit thought she couldn't come out and say the hard thing, not to mention she had already been a cancer survivor and was living life in the program. I looked up to Brit. She opened up to me about sleeping with Kaden one night and let me in on some things that they shared in their friendship; she wanted to help me better understand Kaden. Brit was totally down with my feelings for Kaden and wanted us to be together, but knew that Kaden would have to decide that on his own. I was willing to wait for this guy and Brit had been my voice of reason. I felt like for the first time in my life, I had a friend who cared about me and my recovery and was doing her part to support her friend, Kaden. After Brit gave me the run-through of Kaden's likes and dislikes, it felt like I had my very own cheat sheet to study. I was already starting to fall in love with what I heard about Kaden.

I was hanging with Brit one night when Kaden called and told her that he needed to meet up with her, eager to share some news about him and Lacy. I didn't know what was going on until I answered my front door after hearing a knock to see Kaden standing in front of me. Yes, a tall, light-skinned man hovered over me, asking if he could come in as I gave him a surprised "Hello." I felt more starstruck by seeing this man than I did when I actually had a 'star' by my side. Kaden walked to my dining room table to meet Brit and spilled some tea about Lacy and their break-up. I followed him to the table where he expressed his enthusiasm for being a free man, giving me the sexiest side smile I had ever seen.

The three of us moved the conversation outside and sat around a firepit that Rupert built in our backyard, talking about why Kaden couldn't stand being with Lacy any longer. I giggled just enough but not too much so he didn't think I was harsh with my opinions of their relationship. As the fire crackled, I stared at Kaden's face and knew that I wanted to give him some space and time to get over Lacy before asking him out. Just as I was about to break out of the trance I was in, Rupert flung open the back door and broke me free from any light-hearted feelings I had going. When Rupert saw Kaden outside, he stomped his way over to me and put his hand around my waist as I stood up to greet him. It was his way of claiming me in front of Kaden, and after all that had gone on in our relationship, I knew Rupert wasn't going to trust my harmless friendship with a handsome man like Kaden.

I told Rupert I was going to walk our guests out and he told me to meet him in the bedroom when I was done. I'm sure he was assuming I was going to come in and jump his bones since it was routine roommate shit, but instead, I followed my instincts since my heart longed for something different. I decided to give Britani and Kaden a ride down my long driveway to their car and gave Britani a nod goodnight as she got out.

Kaden was in my passenger seat when he looked at me and softly said, "Thank you for tonight," and I gave him the softest look of contentment, replying "Anytime." Before Kaden opened the car door, he asked me if he could kiss me. I wasted no time answering and leaned into his nose and said yes. I felt his soft lips touch mine with such passion, such strength, behind his intention for that kiss that it forced my eyes to stay shut. I had always been a peaky kisser with people, eyes fluttering to stay open just enough to see the person kissing me. I had never felt so safe in a kiss before. I knew he meant no harm or disrespect for acting so soon. For the first time in my romantic life, I felt a sense of security with the touch of a man. Kaden's kiss gave me such strong pressure throughout my whole body that I sat in my driver's seat, stunned well after he left. I put my car in drive and went back into the house to break up with Rupert for a final time.

Within days of sharing our first kiss, I managed to get Rupert kicked out of our place so I could have Kaden over as often as he was available. He lived 45 minutes away in the same town Brit lived in, so it was convenient to have my two favorite people carpool to my place to visit. Kaden and I spent our time getting to know each other by being barricaded indoors since a global pandemic had taken over the world as we knew it. All of our NA meetings were hosted on Zoom and any new friendships that were formed were strictly virtual and short-lived. It was a strange time to say the least but Kaden and I didn't feel the effects of our city locked down one bit. We were happy to be wrapped up in each other as the world went up in flames. As addicts, we shared the common belief that we could die at any moment, so we should live life to the fullest. But as a Christian, I wanted Kaden to know that I had finally found a higher power that took authority over my life, and I wanted to share that kind of love with him. A structured love.

To find something, outside of people, that pushed a healthy perspective for me was rare, especially when I was an emotional wreck. I began to see the welfare of my mental health when my discipline to meditate and dig into scripture was at the top of my priority list. No one, not even myself, could save me from the wreckage of my accidents, and putting my Christian faith at the center of my life was the best I could do at the time, sacrificing "fun" in order to reap the benefits of a peaceful life. Longevity and peace were my main concerns, and I waited my whole life for something that would last versus a temporary fix. My illness had me wavering all my capabilities. I used to believe the lie that I couldn't accomplish anything my heart most desired, and fear was the result of my lie. I had to sacrifice fear if I was truly going to let God show me who He was and who I was through Him.

I never understood the term 'Born Again Christian' until I chose to identify as a Christ follower and took my baptismal date as my birth date. To be a Christian was to be born again, and what I was taught was that the transformation I would go through would be just like a real birth. I would go from being a baby Christian, with fresh eyes and a new spirit, to a teenage Christian who rebels and fights the process of God's plan for my life, to the adult Christian who can not unknow Him after witnessing His hand in my life. It was getting harder and harder for me to deny the love I was feeling when I walked closely with God and I wanted Kaden to walk with me. I wanted to make room for what was to come instead of trying to predict my own life all the time. Kaden made me want to surrender to God that much more so I could prove that I had it in me to make our relationship work, and that I could keep my eyes fixed on him and only him. I knew I couldn't do it alone.

Kaden wasn't raised in a religious home but was influenced by pagan beliefs from his mom and dad, which I had no problem with. I had been dubbed a gypsy in my family. Still, I wanted us to enthrall ourselves with the same belief system as Christians. The loving ones, might I add. I had known that my pride had gotten in the way of a lot in my life, and if I was going to spare myself from repeated mistakes, then I would have to stay close to my Christianity. This meant church groups, like-minded friends, and Biblical values. Living by my pride was my way of telling God I didn't need Him and I was ready to chip away at my pride each chance I got. I told myself "I'm here for it," knowing that Kaden was willing to join the congregation with me and devote his heart to loving Jesus Christ as well. This wasn't like the first time I joined the church with Leo, having to combat his resistance to the Christian faith. This was a whole new approach with a man who was willing to join the church with an open heart. Kaden and I had a serious conversation one night about my values for my life moving forward, and I discussed some expectations I had if we were going to take things to the next level—something I had never done before.

I told Kaden I wanted a man who had the gusto to chase God the way I had been chasing him at the time, even though I was still making poor decisions like playing dirty by kicking Rupert out of the house. I knew I wanted to try harder to be a woman of my word and not just live to get what I wanted, to instead live for others and feel alive by learning a different type of love. The type of love that isn't boastful or punishing. The love that doesn't just freely give away my body but is patient and genuine. I had made Kaden wait before we slept together and it was mind-blowing how receptive he was to my challenge. I remember testing the waters by arousing him and leading him to take a drink before I took the cup away and told him that no matter how thirsty he was, I wasn't going to give him a sip. He was totally fine with it! I had never experienced such tolerance from a man as I did with Kaden; it was always "Don't leave me with blue balls!" or "Can you at least give me a blow job?" Kaden was respectful and it was beautiful. I knew I could trust him and he didn't make me feel guilty for walking away from our heated moments, so I knew that when we finally did have sex, it was going to be special.

Kaden and I had been dating for a couple of months before I woke up from a nap one day with the most intense feeling of suspicion. Out of nowhere, I opened my eyes gratingly as if I were a robot that had just rebooted. I had been in a deep sleep on my couch when I felt the need to call out for Kaden. There was no response in the house, and I knew he was going to take the dogs for a walk along the river that was right behind my backyard, but I was confused as to why they weren't back yet. Worry fell over me and I rushed to put my shoes on to go find him. I had tried to call his phone as I hiked down to the river but there was no answer. When I got to the bottom of the stream I looked left, then right, and saw nothing. I was having an out-of-body experience, or maybe it was God, but something told me to go right and follow the trail upstream. I began to power walk over rocks and sand, doing my best to avoid the water, when I saw a neon stripe in the distance.

I started to run towards the leash that had been swinging in the air when I noticed it was Kaden walking with my dog, Aztec. I lit up with excitement to see them both and when Kaden saw me running towards him, he splashed his way towards me as fast as he could. We met in the middle of the river and stood on a shallow rock when he grabbed my face and kissed me. I told him how my nap was abruptly interrupted by this strong feeling that I had to come find him and that's when Kaden pulled out a small box from his pocket, opening it before I could finish my sentence. Small raindrops started to fall on my face as I looked up at Kaden with a smile and asked him if he was serious.

Kaden grabbed my chin after pulling the ring out of the box and asked "Will you marry me?" and without hesitation, I confidently said "YES!" I said yes without a worry in my mind or doubt in my heart. I said yes for the first time and actually meant it. As we walked back home, we skipped and danced with so much joy that even the dog was vibing with our blissful mood.

It was time to move in together. Even though I knew that every time I roomed with my lover it had ended badly, Kaden was different. I knew there was a reason the Bible states clear boundaries for marriage and sex but waiting until we were married before having sex and living together didn't seem feasible. I thought that since it was the 21st century and I was turning my life around, our situation was the exception. I wish I had learned more about God's word and what he had intended for my life before it was too late. I'm sure you've heard it said that if you want to make God laugh, tell him your plans. I told God my plans, down to the very detail of wanting to introduce Kaden to my dad and tell him that we planned on having a baby together.

Kaden wrote all over his truck "She said yes!" with shoe polish and paraded our new engagement around town. I had briefly felt horrible for Rupert and how things ended, but then remembered how he slapped me right before we broke up, and I was back to feeling fine with announcing our engagement to everyone. One of the first people I told was Brit and they were thrilled! Brit was just about to get a double mastectomy and faced their fears of coming out as trans to Kaden so it seemed that everyone had a reason to celebrate. I was about to marry my dream man, my window man, and try for a baby! Kaden had already had one child with an ex-girlfriend and I was fully accepting of it. It almost served as a backup plan for me if I couldn't carry another baby to term and risk disappointing Kaden. He made it known that he wanted more kids but he wanted to have them after he found his wife and now—there I was. I had been getting positive reports from my Endocrinologist about my T1D, so I felt like my body and mind were in the right place; not to mention the everlasting pressure from my mom about my age and that if I was going to have children I better "get on it." No pun intended.

Life was going according to plan and after Kaden met Lars, we mailed out engagement party invites the next day. My dad agreed to host the festivities for us, which I was relieved about since after our walk down the aisle last time didn't end very well. I knew my dad was doing his best to support me by keeping his opinions and judgments to himself. After all, he knew I would spot the hypocrisy of him telling me not to follow through with a third marriage. Even if he had told me that my decision to get married and have a baby with someone I just met wasn't the right move to make, would I have listened? I knew how fast I was moving; it's what I'd always done. I wasn't sure at the time if it was resilience, or if I was just crazy in love for wanting to do all of this again.

I used to believe that the greatest gift you could give a man was a baby. I wanted to do something so magnificent for my and Kaden's life that the only thing that would suffice was his DNA combined with mine to make the perfect child. Surely, it would ensure the extent of my love for him by bearing his child even though we hadn't been together long. I thought it was the ultimate act of devotion to help secure our marriage. It's not like I wasn't aware of how backward I was going about things, but I never followed the rules, so who cared about going in chronological order? I just wanted what I wanted, and my love addiction had proven no different than my sex addiction in the sense that my need for validation was in demand and feeling "good" was the end game. Happiness was just a baby delivery away from our new lives together as a blended family, and Kaden was my perfect match to finally see things through to the end.

My dad's property held every guest and dance move until late at night. The DJ had been on fire with the specific set list I had chosen for Kaden and he knew how music was one of my love languages. I'll always remember the time Kaden showed me one of his favorite songs and held up his arm for me to see the goosebumps that caused his air to stand up and I knew in that moment, that Kaden was the guy for me. Kaden had never enjoyed parties growing up because he never really had them, and after his dad died when he was 13, he lost any desire to celebrate anything, especially for himself. Kaden hadn't been speaking to his mom, Karen, over the last year for multiple reasons, but the biggest one was her inability to respect Kaden the way he deserved to be respected. Karen was another one of those surrogate-spouse mothers who projected all of her life trauma onto her son, expecting him to perform to her caliber, and when he didn't, she shunned him and made him earn back her love. I would know how to identify such a character since I thought it was my job to take on those roles, not the mother of my lover.

Our engagement gave me the right to reach out to Karen and introduce myself to her as her son's fiancé. She hadn't known that I was a serial dater looking for her king on the chessboard, or who I was and where I came from, so it took her coming to our party to find out. Karen had written Kaden off after a custody battle over Kaden's daughter, and other selfish reasons, leaving the two of them estranged. I understand there are two sides to every story but I only cared about Kaden's side. He was honest with me about his past and I accepted him for it. At the end of the day, I stand firm that if Karen was the parent, then she should assume her position as one and Kaden as the son. I believe parents are allowed to make mistakes but should never abandon a child who makes it known they want a relationship with said parent. In no way is it ok for a parent to behave like the child when, in fact, the child is in need of a loving, tender parent. This core belief sprouted once I saw the reality of my own home life, so finding the male version of myself in Kaden had me wanting to mend his open wounds.

Once Karen read my FB message about coming back together with Kaden to celebrate our lives, she was able to show up to our party long enough to see how happy he was and how his life was moving in a brighter direction. Like most parents of addicts, Karen was skeptical about how long Kaden's sobriety was going to last; no different than her thoughts about our marriage. Looking back, I can't blame her for that, but I did blame her for how she tortured the man I loved for most of his life as Kaden opened up about his mom and how she treated him after his dad died. I had no idea what pain Kaden had been living with until he released it in the worst way. Just when you think that you want your love life to be a scene out of a rom-dram (romantic-drama) movie, you come to your senses and pray that you get a different life outside of something scripted and manipulated for entertainment. For the first time in my life, I knew I didn't want my romantic relationship to be for my amusement. I wanted to protect my home life for the sake of my child's future because Kaden and I were pregnant!

A month after our party and bookoo[1] sex sessions, Kaden and I hit the mark with what I believe did the trick. I was beginning to worry that I wasn't going to conceive and Kaden did everything to track my ovulation; he even made me stop using vagina wash in the shower because he thought that the ingredients would prevent his sperm from reaching an egg. I settled the dispute after a shower session one day by twerking upside on him and letting his sperm really reach up in me to find my eggs. I could've sworn it was that time because three weeks later, I was crying to Kaden about the positive pregnancy test. I was triggered and panicked and told Kaden I regretted the decision we

_____

[1] Slang meaning in great quantity or a lot of

made to try once I found out. I felt like the baby was going to die on me again and we should just prepare for the worst. Kaden had no idea how to handle my hormones or my trauma triggers other than to shut down. Everything I had ever experienced in relationships was repeating itself in that moment and I didn't know what to do.

Kaden had his medical marijuana card and he always took to puffing when scenarios like this would break out. I was doing absolutely everything to abstain from any mind-altering substances in fear that I would relapse and lose all my sobriety all over again. Four years had passed since my last sip of alcohol or drug use, and I wasn't going to let anything make me relapse, not even Kaden. Kaden and I were still active in the NA program and I wanted him to eventually be where I was at - fully clear-headed without the crutch of drugs, with years under his belt. I believe in the power of medicinal marijuana, but to me, there is a fine line between it being medicine or it being a drug. Kaden had only been sober for a few days from using alcohol and other illicit drugs right before I met him and it was our mutual friend, Evan, that led him to the rooms of NA. Kaden was a hot mess, about to sleep with his first hooker, when Evan intervened and brought him to a meeting in Fanta Se, where I met him. Even though Kaden was approaching his nine-month mark of sobriety from alcohol and drugs, I was still having trouble trusting him with how to control his marijuana usage. I had known of the hole he was in before he came into my life, since my hole was identical, but I hadn't known the extent of his torment until it was too late.

After making sure our pregnancy was in the safe zone with reassurance from our doctor that I would carry to term, Kaden and I decided to shout on top of a mountain that we were pregnant! I wasn't going to let my traumatic past define this pregnancy, and I was over the moon about being a mother. I felt like I had all my bases covered with medical care by seeing a gang of specialists for both my physical and mental health. I'll never forget my therapist asking me if I was ready to NOT be the center of attention anymore. During one of our sessions, I admitted how I was relieved to know that a child was going to be my focus now and all the attention I had been getting was soon to be shifted onto a new life. I felt ready for it! It was what came after the pregnancy glow that I wasn't ready for.

Kaden and I had been watching Sage Church online since the doors weren't open yet to the public in our city. The pandemic forced us to stay in front of a screen, and that meant inviting loved ones over to share a church service with us. I loved hosting friends and loved ones to share church services and a warm meal. Now that Kaden had custody over his daughter again, things really felt like home. Even Brit had joined in for church services, and as Kaden introduced me to each of his friends, I felt it was an opportunity to invite them to church. I had learned that the power of being a believer was held in knowing Christ and making Christ known, and it would appear that I had a niche for bringing people to church. Something of an evangelist, and I thoroughly enjoyed it.

It was the end of summer and fall was approaching when Kaden told me about an old friend of his named Hunter and how he wanted to make plans to meet up with him since they hadn't seen each other over the last year. I had wondered why Hunter wasn't at our engagement party after listening to Kaden explain to me the magnitude of their friendship. I told myself I wasn't going to have any sexual thoughts about my fiancé's friends, and I exercised that after meeting all of the guy friends in Kaden's life. As we were on our way to meet Hunter at a coffee shop, Kaden unpacked some facts about Hunter, and the things he had to tell me were slightly unsettling to say the least. Kaden's daughter, Kelly, sat next to me at a table in a small courtyard while Kaden grabbed our food and drinks when I heard the revving of a motorcycle pull up. Under normal circumstances, I'd be all over my boyfriend's best friend, but for once I had no intention of picturing myself with anyone besides Kaden.

Just as Kaden sat our drinks down, Hunter took off his helmet and walked over to hug Kaden. I noticed Kelly's face lit up like a star on a Christmas tree when Hunter bent over to hug her hello. I stood up to shake his hand and introduced myself when I saw tattoos peak through his long-sleeved shirt; I thought to myself, "No wonder this guy shot someone, he's got bad boy written all over him," and with the smell of cigarettes lingering on his clothes, I immediately felt sick at the idea of picking up a cigarette again. I nodded and smiled along to the stories they shared with one another and couldn't help but think of how much I loved Kaden and Kelly that even someone who was typically my type, like Hunter, couldn't tempt me. I knew judging Hunter was the safest thing for me to do because I didn't want any of Kaden's past friendships derailing all the hard work he had been putting in towards his new life. I had even asked Brit to back off a bit from getting high or sharing weed with Kaden to ensure his recovery was the top priority.

We all bonded and enjoyed the afternoon together when my guard came down just enough to allow Hunter to reunite with his best friend after being released from jail. Kelly and Kaden both loved him, and considering how long Hunter had been a part of their lives, I had better get used to him being around too. From what I learned, Hunter had been sober and working on himself, which was good for me because I wanted nothing to do with anyone using around me; I was toxic enough on my own. I knew I could act out by flaunting myself in front of Hunter but I was determined to fight for the loyalty I had never seen growing up, felt in my dating life, or earned by living a clean life from substance abuse. Kaden was my first love I felt I wanted to try for– work for. I wanted him to be my last, and I looked at him like he was a bee amongst flies, and Hunter— Hunter was a wasp. I couldn't let Hunter be a part of our lives without inviting him to church, so the following weekend he joined us for an in-home sermon - which was the last time I saw Hunter until he reappeared in my life when I least expected it.

Chapter 13

#triggered

A fight broke out between my brothers Blake and Jax at my dad's house one evening during a family gathering, leaving Kaden disappointed with my dad. Enough to call Lars up and ask him what the hell he was thinking. I had never had a man defend me before like Kaden did. He called my dad and asked him why he allowed Blake's girlfriend to harass me while I was four months pregnant, asking why the hell he didn't step in to protect me while I was being ganged up on by my stepbrother's wife while my stepmother stood by and gossipped. Shiela had always struggled with me for one reason or another and no matter how hard we tried to like each other, we always fell short. My dad simply responded to Kaden with a drunk tongue:

"You don't know me Kaden, and I think it's best you just stay out of it."

"I can't stay out of it; my fiancé is pregnant and I find it unacceptable that you would let such violence take place around her. I'm pissed that you didn't do anything but stand there while chaos erupted!"

"Kaden, I'm done. I don't owe you anything. I'm hanging up the phone now."

Kaden had been at work while I was at my dad's for a family celebration, and Kaden hadn't been a part of our family long enough to see the dysfunction of cruelty that always took place. Jax was in and out of jail constantly, stirring the pot with his dick by sleeping with every one of my friends, and Blake hated me for not liking his girlfriend and being the child that got her way while he went by, barely noticed. Not to mention my stepbrother Brandon who was infatuated with me to the point of not wanting to give up making sexual passes at me. It seemed like the only one left to look at was my dad. Lars was the biggest coward of them all in my eyes because he never could bring himself to apologize or acknowledge his behavior.

My dad blocked me and Kaden after he hung up on Kaden, and I was right back where I started with him all because my fiancé wasn't going to be intimidated by his superiority but I loved Kaden for that. I couldn't believe I was back on radio silence with my dad. Now that I was pregnant, I needed him more than ever. Things began to spiral as my pregnancy progressed and I felt hopeless not having my dad or my mom nearby. Kaden was working as much as he could to financially prepare for the baby. When he expressed his concerns about money, I assured him that we were going to be okay and that perhaps we should go camping to take his mind off things. Kaden loved the outdoors and helped me be active during my depressive states through the hormone fluctuation. We were happy when we were alone together and everyone saw it, including Kaden's ex-girlfriends.

After our camping trip to the mountains, Kaden began to shift his perspective about affording this new baby and was beginning to get excited! We were baby shopping and rearranging our house to prepare for him/her, and since we were awaiting our ultrasound appointment, we didn't know if we were having a boy or a girl. I had a feeling I was having a boy, so I told Kaden I wanted to focus on picking out boy names. We both agreed on the name being of Viking descent since Kaden had the bloodline. He opened up to me about his father's lineage and how he wanted our son to have a strong name like his father. That's when Kaden told me a strange story about his father's passing. Kaden was torn when he got the news as a young teen that he lost his father in a car accident. But what Kaden hadn't told anyone, until he found out more about what happened as an adult, was that he believed his father purposely crashed the car. Committing suicide. I cried when he shared his father's love for his mother but that Karen wasn't in a place for forgiveness and refused to take Kaden's father back. The story of their separation was all too familiar and of course, Karen had her own story of what happened, but again, all that mattered was how my fiancé felt about this titanic loss.

Just when Kaden was sharing his process of grieving his father, we got a phone call that our friend Evan died from a purposeful drug overdose. Evan had taken his life right after his ex-girlfriend left him. We agreed that we would never really know why he died, but there were strong indications of a broken heart. To me, a broken heart consists of many pieces, and what I've learned from experience is that we women are a huge component. Kaden and I had just attended Evan's funeral when Kaden's business partner called him asking for his help because his roommate had just shot himself with a 22 rifle. Death was everywhere caused by the pandemic, and the rates of suicide were climbing. I was starting to feel the effects of the aftermath and it was somber. I was unaware that a 22-caliber rifle could actually kill a person, and that's when Kaden responded with the most disturbing response.

"Yeah, Lovey, a 22 bullet is a perfect bullet to get the job done because if you shoot yourself in the head it will ping-pong around in your skull, making sure you don't ever survive."

Jax was back in jail, Brit wasn't speaking to me after my request to keep away from Kaden, and my dad had bailed on me again. My pregnancy glow had died out after all the drama and Kaden had been struggling to process his emotions around the one friend who led him to his sobriety. He was a mess. There would be nights he would come home from work and didn't eat, and his sleep pattern was disrupted by his anxiety, causing his mental and physical health to decline. Kaden and I had been fighting in ways I had never experienced with him before and I slowly grew paranoid. I could see that Kaden would take his aggression or pent up emotions out on me by having sex, and though it wasn't violent/rough sex, I felt it being used as a weapon. I could always spot my own behaviors, more specifically those involving sex, and I knew my fiancé was a sex addict in addition to being bisexual. I thought I could help him find solace in his wound-up mind but no amount of pegging could get Kaden right. He was on the cusp of relapsing to cope.

I was an emotional basket case one evening after receiving a letter from Jax and called to cry to my mom about how hurt I was to know he was writing me from jail. I had been heartbroken over so many things and the joy of my pregnancy was non-existent at that point. While I was on the phone, Kaden came home from work and saw me in the living room crying as my mom walked me through my anxiety attack. I gave him the famous 'one sec' finger as I cried out to my mom about how miserable I was with all my heavy emotions. When I finally calmed down to take a few deep breaths, I hung up the phone after telling my mom I loved her. I wiped my face and walked to our bedroom to see that Kaden changed out of his work clothes and was sitting on our bed with a 22 rifle in his hands.

"Babe, what are you doing?"

"You're not happy."

"What do you mean? Yes, I am. I'm just having a hard time and my mom talked me through it. What is that? Where did you get that rifle?"

"It was my dad's. He gave it to me."

I walked over to the bed where Kaden was sitting with the erect rifle and tried to touch it but he gripped it tighter and pulled it away from me. I looked at Kaden and he began to cry without opening his eyes.

"Baby, what's wrong? Why are you crying? I know we got into a fight earlier but everything is going to be ok."

Silence.

"Kaden?"

I started to panic all over again when I noticed Kaden wasn't responding to me. I sat close to him and tried to turn his face towards me when he resisted. I pulled my phone out when Kaden's eyes sprung open and he looked at me with an emptiness I'd never seen before. His blue eyes turned black and he quickly snatched my phone out of my hands and asked me who I was calling before I even had a chance to unlock it.

I told him, "No one, I was just checking my blood sugar," since I had an app that constantly monitored my levels. Kaden demanded me not to contact anyone, and that's exactly when I knew I needed to call for help. He had fallen off the deep end and was acting crazy. I didn't take it seriously at first until he began crying again and I sat in front of him, trying to take the rifle away when he yanked it back and scooted over to the other side of the bed.

"Kaden, please give me the rifle and just hold me."

Silence.

"Or let's call your mom - my mom helped me through my hard time!"

"My mom doesn't care. Nothing I did was ever good enough, why would she care now? She's a bitch to me, she's always been a bitch to me."

"Then let's call Brit! We can get through whatever you're feeling. Let me hold you."

I did my best to cuddle up next to Kaden while he sat up against our headboard and held the rifle tighter than any grip he had ever had on me. I pleaded with him while his eyes stayed shut and tears ran down his face. I didn't know what else to do other than let him be in hopes it would pass. I managed to catch some blurry photos of Kaden holding the rifle by pretending to check my glucose levels while I got up and walked to our spare bathroom across the house. I sat on the toilet and was hoping to send the photos to Brit so she would rush over, but Kaden appeared in the doorway and asked what I was doing. I was startled to see him but somewhat relieved knowing he got out of the room when I answered, "Nothing, just going pee."

Kaden watched me wipe and kept an eye on my phone as I picked up my PJ shorts and walked out of the bathroom. I turned around and asked Kaden if we could go to bed already since it had been well passed my bedtime but he answered with an icy "No."

Kaden went back to the bedroom and sat on his side of the bed when I told him that I wanted to go to sleep and turned off the lights. Kaden reached over, turned them back on, and closed his eyes as he sat up clenching the 22. I was boiling inside that Kaden was acting this way so I tried to reach for the rifle again when he pulled it away from me, this time whispering to me "Please stop." His calm manner had me so freaked out that I sat on his lap, facing him, begging him to open his eyes.

He opened his eyes and tears poured like waterfalls down to his shirt. I began to sob with him. I told Kaden I loved him, and whatever he was thinking, he could let it go, that he didn't have to go through with it. I managed to break one of his hands free from the rifle and held it to my belly, shouting at him "Don't do this to us! Why are you doing this?! Don't you love us?!" Kaden pulled his hand back into his torso to hold the rifle closer this time. I thought I could take the rifle away from him if he started to fall asleep, but there was no sleeping. Kaden and I sat up in our bed, wrestling his demons for hours, before I finally asked him the question that had been on my mind:

"Are you going to kill me?"

"Please, just go."

My internal monologue kept repeating that if we made it out alive, I was going to leave him for doing this to me. The level of terror I felt for losing my life had me so numb, I was calm. The saying *there's always a calm before the storm* was proven to be true at that moment, and it was like Kaden knew what I was thinking; he knew he was going to lose me whether or not he pulled the trigger.

I slowly got off the bed and walked towards our spare bedroom when I fainted. I was out—cold. I had never fainted before so I wasn't sure how long you were supposed to be out for, but being pregnant and diabetic on top of going through stress as a hostage to my loved one had my body at its limit. I woke up to see the sun through the window and I looked at my phone that was right beside me. It read 6:12 AM. I walked across the living room since I hadn't made it that far from our bedroom. I walked in to see blood splatter on the sheets and Kaden's body folded over on our bed in the same spot I last saw him. I bolted out of the doorway of our room and ran across the house to our spare bedroom where I jumped out of the window. I landed on the gravel and still had my phone in my hand when I dialed 911 with a shaky hand. It was chilly outside as I screamed and cried, waiting for red and blues to show up and give me a sense of comfort. Red and blues aren't known to comfort people, but on October 12, 2020, they were my saving grace.

I was shivering in my shorts and cut-off T-shirt as two units and an ambulance pulled up to the house. The EMTs quickly noticed I was going into shock and put me into the back of the ambulance to take care of me. The officer on the scene did his best to wait it out while I came to so he could question me about what happened. Have you ever tried to speak to someone while they are in a state of hysteria? It doesn't fucking work! The medics instructed the officers to meet us at the hospital as they drove off while I sat upright on the gurney, feeling nothing but the vibrations of my heart tearing through my body. First, it was silent like when you hold your fingers over your ears. Then it was loud like I needed headphones just to stabilize myself. The only thing I could think to do was call Rupert. I couldn't call my dad to come meet me at the hospital, and my mom was in TX, but I knew Rupert and my dad were still speaking since that's just what dad does. So when Rupert answered the phone all I could say was, "Kaden's dead. I need you to call my dad for me and tell him to call me."

Rupert began to cry the second he heard those fatal words leave my mouth and through my whimpering, he told me that he would call my dad right away and hung up the phone. I'll always love Rupert for answering the phone, for the love he did show me after all I had done to him, especially through our break-up, he still let me in when I knocked. My heart stung with such strong grief that I felt more abandoned than ever before, by my dad and now by Kaden. Was it me? Did Kaden die because of something I did or didn't do? All I could do was question myself before making another phone call to Kristi since I knew that she would be the one to come rescue me. My mom and dad never cared to show support for my downfalls unless it was something dramatic like a hospital visit; never mind remembering the hell I went through with my disease on a daily or showing support for how sick I'd been throughout the years. All I wanted was consistent, subtle support as I trekked through life, but what I got was their selfishness until the story was too big for them to ignore. I arrived at the hospital and was wheeled to the E.R. where I was evaluated by nurses before calling my mom to tell her what happened.

How else are you supposed to deliver the news about your fiancé's death other than bluntly? As soon as my mom gathered a sentence, she hung up the phone and headed towards NM to come get me. I was told by a nurse that after my psych evaluation, if I passed, I'd get to go home, but they would only release me to a family member. As I sat up in the hospital bed, kicking my legs back and forth in a slow, bicycle-like manner, a detective walked in and noticed that I was still crying. He told me he would come back in 20 minutes to give me some time to pull it together - as if 20 minutes was all I needed. It would be five hours before my mom would arrive, so I frantically scrolled through my contacts to see which friend of mine could come to be with me while I waited, to keep me from pulling the plug on myself. It's scary to think about placing yourself in the same position as your dead lover, and that's exactly what was happening to me. I didn't want to spread the news about Kaden, but I was terrified of being alone in a hospital with such images burned in my brain.

After I had a friend hold me by my bedside while I wept, the detective came back and gave me the "it's time" look. So, I listened to every question he had for me and I answered each one so carefully that it was like I had been in that position before. All I did was tell the truth. This time, there was no stretching my story to be in my favor or exaggerating to sound more cool; it was just the sad, ugly truth. I finished the questioning process and handed my phone over to the detective so he could read my messages with Kaden, and that's when

Karen walked into the room. She fell over onto me and began to cry as I went limp and collapsed in her arms with just as much disbelief as she had. When our eyes finally met she wanted to know what happened. I gave her a synopsis of the night, and that's when she asked me "Were you guys fighting?" and BOOM! It hit me. I was going to be to blame for this. Before I could answer her, the detective asked her to step out to speak with him. I went back to curling up in the fetal position before the doctor walked in to give me my psych eval.

My mom helped me out of my wheelchair into the back seat of my grandmother's Mercedes so we could check in at a hotel across the street from the hospital. My Nana had been my mom's travel partner, so it was no surprise when I saw her in the passenger seat. If it weren't for the two of them showing up, I don't think I would have made it through the night. I immediately took a shower when I got into our room and while I sat on the bleached white, tiled floor, I held my belly in fear that I hurt the baby with all the stress my body went through. I wanted to get an ultrasound as soon as possible to make sure the worst wasn't happening. I couldn't stand the thought of losing the baby too, but before I reached for my phone to call my doctor, a black and white photo of me and my dad popped up as it rang on the bathroom counter. I was irate but I wanted to talk to him more than anything so I answered. It dawned on me that listening to my dad's voice on the other end of a phone call with a lump in my throat was no different than all the relationships I shared with men who caused that lump. There was no time to hash out our issues; I just needed him to comfort me any way he could.

After my father gave his tears of condolence and his promise that he would be available to me, night and day, it didn't matter, I started to feel my body coming to a calm after all the adrenaline spikes I was getting. He assured me that we were going to get through this tragedy together, and I actually believed him that time. I got off the phone with Lars and my phone would not stop ringing with calls from friends and NA members, including Kaden's sponsor who I despised with every fiber of my being. After Arnold sent Kaden a dick pic and professed his undying crush on him, I knew the guy was no good, but I answered his call anyway. If anyone was going to spread a story like I used to spread my legs, it was Arnold. After giving him the rundown, I answered only one other person's call before my mom told me to put my phone away and get some rest. It felt impossible to turn it off, and all I wanted was to spew what had happened to me. Each time I delivered my truth, it felt more and more true.

After a night of broken sleep, I walked across the street to get my ultrasound before we packed up to leave to back to Yellow. I knew it was coming, that I was going to end up back at my mom's house, under her watchful eye. I wasn't sure what had me more terrified - having the image of Kaden burned into my brain or living under my mom's roof. There I was, on a medical table, awaiting the news of my unborn child from the sonographer once again, and to my succor, I was told that the baby was just fine and looking textbook healthy. The nurse asked me if I knew the sex of the baby yet. When I told her I didn't, that's when she asked "Do you want to know?" I nodded andshe told me I was having a boy. I cried the whole walk over to the hotel as my mom and Nana loaded up the car. A boy. A beautiful baby boy to carry on Kaden's bloodline. I was so happy yet confused about why I was in this position. How could this happen to me?

As I lay in the back seat of the car, I replayed the entirety of my and Kaden's relationship. What did I miss? They say it's the people who appear the happiest that are the ones struggling the most. I was a moody, happy person, but now that I thought about it, Kaden internalized a lot of his emotions. It was as if he didn't want to express anything other than happiness and there I was, unhappy to my core, thinking that my life was finally perfect but I was alone in the worst way. The only thing I had to distract myself from my very lucid thoughts was my phone. I had so many unopened FB messages and unanswered texts that I started to get a nervous tick from not clicking on them. I decided to reach out to past lovers instead just like some of us do when we try to validate ourselves in hopes past people will resurrect our spirit. I messaged Ara and Micah and checked in with Rupert. I had thought about reaching out to Leo, but after I wrote him an amends letter when I first started going to NA, I promised myself I would leave him alone. Maybe it was because of how fragile he was when it came to me - he almost died because of me. Or was it me? Did I kill Leo with my love? Did I kill Zieya by not loving her? Was I really the reason Kaden's dead?

Have you ever felt so angry you were afraid that it would be permanent? I have. I was in a place that had me in a headlock, preventing me from breathing, and no matter how calm I remained, I was going to fade out into death. Lifeguards are told to teach swimmers not to panic when they are treading water and to do their best not to drown. I felt like I was ready to drown. My lungs were filling with water whether I stayed calm or not. I couldn't breathe and the only thing keeping me alive was the rage inside; the fight to stay alive. I was choosing anger and hurt simultaneously because that's what made sense to me. The two are gay for each other, and it was important for me to know they both existed, kind of like the anomaly of what came first, the chicken or the egg? Was my anger born out of hurt? Or was my hurt born out of anger? All I knew was that I wanted to escape my reality like never before.

I'd been tormented throughout my life and all I wanted was to erase it from my mind; what better way than drugs and alcohol? I was reliving emotions and situations that I didn't think I would ever have to again, and I could only assume that that was the thing about letting your guard down—it was always too soon. I shouldn't have been surprised by the drama that unfolded, being that it felt like I was destined for trauma, but I really had hopes for my life and thought I was done living in sadness. I thought I was out of the thick of it when my sorrow declared that I needed to relapse and take my life. I had been prescribed Lorazepam by a doctor before I left the hospital, and my mom was instructed on how I needed to handle the highly addictive drug. I had been speaking to Rupert every chance I got the moment I arrived in TX and told him I wanted to take the whole bottle so I could end my suffering. Rupert was concerned for me and wanted to be available to help me deal. Part of that looked like him ratting me out to my mom about my suicide craving.

Every time I'd wanted to die it was interrupted by my selfish thinking. "What if I don't get to do this or what if I don't get to do that?" Pure FOMO[1]. It was always "I" "I" "I" when it came to my moments of thinking about taking my life, which in hindsight was a good thing, but I wondered if that was what Kaden was thinking when he aimed and fired. I think it was the complete opposite because Kaden was the least selfish person I knew. He should have been more selfish if it meant keeping his life. Just as I was about to down the whole bottle of pills, my mom walked through my bedroom door and made sure it wasn't going to happen. Why couldn't I just get this done? Did I need a gun? I cried myself to sleep that night and slept like I was dead, with no recollection of what happened before I was out. The amnesia had

---

[1] FOMO = fear of missing out

kicked in after my first night in my old bedroom. Then it was delirium before denial, and I was well on my way through all the seven stages of grief: shock, denial, anger, bargaining, depression, testing, and acceptance. There were some moments I experienced all at once, and lest we forget that I'd done this before, I was stacking all my previous trauma-grief on my current trauma like a game of Jenga.

Before I left NM, Karen had gone over to my and Kaden's house to pack me a bag since I couldn't stomach walking into our bedroom with the blood-stained sheets and the desolate feeling of the torture. It was in our bedroom that Karen found a binder with multiple suicide notes in it that Kaden had written to various people, me being one of them. Mine read:

> Dear Lovey,
>
> I know that I have burdened you with my past and it seems like it's all too much. I never wanted to hurt you or make you feel like you had to carry all my weight. I promised I would do anything to protect you and I am so scared to go back out and relapse again. You are stronger than I am and the most beautiful person I've ever met. You are everything to me. I love you. Take care of our baby.

It wasn't until a family member of Kaden's sent me a picture of the handwritten note via text message that I started to feel like it wasn't my fault that Kaden left me behind with his unborn child. I wanted to look at him like he was a monster for what he put me through that fateful night, but then I remembered the face that stared me in the eyes every morning, asking for my hand in prayer - that was the true Kaden Riley. God knows sick, and Kaden was nothing short of sick—but so was his mother. Karen called me three days after his death, screaming at me that it was my fault he died. She asked me why I didn't wrestle the gun away from him since my dad was a cop and I should have known how to handle someone with a gun. Karen then decided to threaten me by telling me that she was going to come after me and put a bullet through my head after what happened to her poor Kaden. And just like that, I was back to feeling like everything was my fault.

Once Karen hung up on me, I let my pain and shame out through my tears as I sat and contemplated what to do next. I told my mom what Karen said and my mom advised me to keep my distance from her. I did one better and filed a police report. I wanted so badly to fight dirty, to get back at her for what she said, and I knew that she was grieving like I was, but she took it too far when she lashed out blaming me. It was through FB and word of mouth that I found out about Karen slandering my name. She took to social media and posted a video with her husband about how I was a danger, a threat to society, and how I was the one who killed Kaden; that I was the one who shot him. My Facebook was flooded with shared posts about how I was trash, the devil incarnate, and how I should be in jail for what I did to Kaden. The cyberbullying was real and didn't stop there. Kaden's baby mama called me and told me she was going to open a case against me and have me thrown in jail for assisted suicide. While screaming at me, she blamed my Christian faith for why Kaden died. She told me that Kaden had never believed in God and he was fine his whole life but now that I forced him to follow Christianity, he went crazy and couldn't stand it. The atrocity that was that conversation was beyond me. I wanted to use all of my defense mechanisms to control my situation by pulling all my strings to go after Karen and the other trolls for kicking me while I was down, but instead, I fawned and prayed.

When detectives called me to assure me that it was a clear suicide by Kaden's hand and there was no way I could go to jail, I sighed a shallow breath of relief. Knowing that everyone was blaming me for this death had me going through mental strain that only God could get me through. God and Rupert. And a dating app. My dad was doing his job by walking me through the hardest parts of my night terrors by relating with me over a common terror of seeing dead bodies. Rupert was my sense of love that I needed to get me through the abandonment I felt from Kaden; he was my cushion. Then there were the dating apps to ensure I had my sex on standby. As if the death of my dream boy wasn't enough, his mother and everyone who knew him were out to get me while I lay in bed pregnant, suffering from COVID-19. I had finally caught the virus when I got to TX and felt like I was going to die. Finally, my time had come! I was back in a hospital bed, ready for the virus to kill my baby boy and myself, when doctors told me that if it weren't for the baby inside of me, the virus probably would have taken my life with the gravity of my autoimmune disease. God must've really wanted me to survive for some unknown reason, so it was time to pick myself up and walk toward my healing....whatever that looked like.

After a couple of dates and a hook-up with the sweetest marine man I'd ever met, I told my mom that it was time to head back to NM to prepare for the baby. I didn't have a penny to my name since Kaden and I had shared everything, and Karen wouldn't even let me have a copy of his death certificate let alone give access to our finances. I wasn't even invited to his funeral, which broke my spirit that much more. I knew there was no showing my face around Kaden's friends or family, but I wanted to go back to Fanta Se so I could be alone to process my emotions. It was when I heard the new rumor that was circulating about me cheating on Kaden and the baby not being his that I finally quit torturing myself and stayed off of FB. I kept my head down and my mouth shut and looked for a way to get back to NM because I had a plan for what I would do once I got there. I wasn't going to let anyone know what I was up to.

Kaden died a week before my 30th birthday, and I told myself that I wasn't going to be 30 and living with my mother as a charity case. Everyone in my family knew what happened to me and it was so hard for me to feel like they weren't treating me differently because of it. Kind of like when someone with cancer finally comes out with their diagnosis and everyone is suddenly nice to them. I wanted my dignity intact as much as possible and losing control over my life was how I found the motivation to make moves. Even the tightest of binds like this couldn't stop me from moving. Trauma did that to me, causing me to not sit still long enough to process, to rest. I wished I would have turned to scripture more. "Be still and know that I am God" (Psalms 46:10) so I wouldn't make the decision I was going to make.

I was going to do anything to prove to my mom that I could make it on my own in Fanta Se, even if that meant blackmailing and manipulating people into helping me. I was a black widowed woman, ready to do whatever it took to go back to a place I considered home. My mom selfishly didn't want me to go and I couldn't be mad at her for always showing up to rescue me. She's always been a mother who made herself physically available for me before she made herself emotionally available, which meant I had to find a way to put a deposit down for my own place because I refused to have her damage add to my already damaged life. I took to asking my therapist for advice and she suggested that I apply for The Empty Stocking Fund. I hate to be cynical but organizations like this thrive off of a dramatic story like mine, and that's exactly what they got when I wrote in my *why* for needing their generous check that holiday season. All I needed was a ride back to Fanta Se, so I asked a friend to come and pick me up, and before you knew it, I was on the road.

Rupert and I had rekindled our flame, like we always did, and he agreed to house me in the very house I kicked him out of until I could find a place to rent. I arrived in Fanta Se and found myself living in fear that I wouldn't be able to find love again, not even with Rupert, if I kept my child. I couldn't drink, smoke, use drugs, or deal. How could I move past the pain of what happened to me? I wanted to believe Rupert agreed to help me because he felt sorry for me, because he loved me. Somewhere along the way, I knew he couldn't pass up an opportunity to finally ejaculate inside of me knowing he couldn't get me pregnant. Plus, he would have access to me whenever he wanted. He had been sleeping with a few other women and had just broken it off with Carla, which I knew was only a matter of time. It was me who had Rupert's heart. He was excited to have me back in his life and back in his bed. He loved how sexy I was with my pregnant belly and something about my hormones made him crazy over me. What Rupert didn't know was that I had planned to abort the baby after making an appointment with a doctor. New Mexico is one of the few states that will abort a child up to eight months in and I was at six.

I called my friends Raven and Bo to drive me to my appointment outside of town while I wrestled with the thought of saying goodbye to the tiny kicks and the turnings on top of my bladder. I felt like this was the way it had to be if I was ever going to find another man to love me and not be alone for the rest of my life. I needed my body back and, most importantly, I needed my sanity back. I didn't feel I could raise a child that resembled Kaden while I stared at him every day with the constant reminder as torture. How could I be a mother now? I was a fucking mess, worse than before, and even though I hadn't relapsed with substances, I had been using sex to cope with my broken heart, again. On my way to the clinic, I let out a few tears since it was all I had left from how much I had been crying. I told Bo to turn off the highway, missing our intended exit, and darted my eyes around looking for a tattoo shop. I needed a fix.

I had Bo drive me to the closest shop with a plan in mind to cover my baby bump under my hoodie. I was overly confident that the artists inside the shop wouldn't notice since all the focus for the tattoo I wanted would go on my face. I had already had a face tattoo on the left side of my cheekbone and above my eyebrow, so this tattoo was going right on my jawline on the right side of my face where I had room. When I shared with Raven and Bo what I was doing, they both replied with encouragement and told me I could do whatever I wanted if it meant canceling my appointment to abort my son. The three of us walked into the shop where I asked a male artist for Kaden's name, pointing to my soft, chubby cheek. He looked at me seriously and replied, "You got it." After staring at the stencil of Kaden's name on my face, I knew I couldn't deny the love I had for him and our child. I wanted his name to stare back at me every day so I could feel like I was still loved by him. I didn't want to abort our baby; I wanted to keep it, and if blasting Kaden's name on my face was my way of diverting from my original decision, then so be it.

I walked out of the shop with more tears coating my face as the burn of the salt stung my tattoo, reminding me of what I had just done. Raven and Bo were so helpful with the way they showed their support that it made some of my family members look bad. I thanked Bo for buying my tattoo and he drove me back to Rupert's where he cradled me all night as he judged my decision for what I did to my "pretty face". He knew my pain was too great to tell me what he thought to my face but I could see it in his. No one wanted to condone my behavior, yet no one wanted to tell me a damn thing about what I was doing. I needed to be saved from myself, and I was remembering that God was the only one who could help me now.

Chapter 14

#thelastdoor

It had been weeks of living back with Rupert when I finally found a small condo that would accept a pregnant, unemployed, trauma victim. It's sad to say how badly I wanted to hide my truth but I knew I had to be honest about my conditions with my renter if I had any shot at being on my own. Lying never positively came full circle, so being transparent was the more reasonable option. It served me well because I got a call about my application being accepted for a one-bedroom condo downtown Fanta Se. Not that I didn't love reliving the good times with Rupert and having his companionship; he was just too much of a reminder of all the bullshit we went through for two years straight. I knew that I couldn't be with him for real even though I exhausted myself trying to. That's the funny thing about the brain, it wants to revert to familiarity. I had let Rupert down just as he had let me down, too many times to count, and it made me feel like I had to try harder for us to work. I was in no position to work hard towards a man, so I made a declaration to focus on nesting and growing my baby once I got into my new place.

Winter had blanketed the town with snow, and as I sat next to my fireplace, I did my best to soak up the essence of being alone. It was always a scary thought to be alone with myself, or my thoughts, so I worked tirelessly to avoid it. It was a full-time job, just like managing my diabetes. Maybe that's what I'd been missing: a chance to meditate on God's word and let Him speak to me without the cloudiness of my thoughts. I had always based my life on how I was feeling, and now it was time to remember that my feelings weren't always right. However, what God says is true, and what is true is that I am loved unconditionally by Him. I can feel without hurting myself or others. I had constantly pushed love away thinking I wasn't worthy of it but now I was in a position that prevented me from pushing back. The thing about God is that you can't push Him, you can do your best to run from Him, but His love will follow you. Everything that had fallen into place with getting my apartment and keeping my child were all blessings I didn't know were God's doing. Every time something good happened to me, I just thought it was because of my control when in reality it was of a higher power. Any time something bad happened, I didn't use it as a tool that it was happening FOR me and I wanted so much to change my perspective on my life. Channeling my grief and anxiety towards God was the best thing for me to get on with my life. That's when I started to cry out WOW is me instead of WOE is me. I knew that I could be happy if I just unpacked my broken heart and worked towards my healing and recovery. It's been said that prayer without work is just prayer.

I was ready to improve my well-being and study up on all the resources available to me as a single mother (rather than a man-eater with status). I wanted to exercise my brain over my beauty and show myself I could take care of business without having to blackmail anyone or fake an interest in someone just to get what I needed. Giving up my power, my pussy power, was one of the hardest reality checks I've ever had. My intention had always been to survive, and I believed the only way to survive as a woman was to flaunt the very thing that made me a woman. It wasn't until God revealed that my power as a woman lay in the depths of my heart that I finally felt accepted for who I was. It's not about being perfect or what my performance claims, but what my heart really desired, cracks and all. What my heart wanted more than anything was to heal from my past and present so I could cope with my future pain better.

After taking a paternity test to prove that my son was, in fact, Kaden's son, I was tempted to clap back at the social media world for ostracizing me. I finally posted a status on my FB page acknowledging what happened with Kaden's death and made sure to keep my words true. I wanted people to know that I wasn't going to react volatilely and instead show that I took some time to choose my words wisely. This is what I wrote:

Monsters. What do you know about them? What I know is that they come out in different forms for each person. The monsters I've seen are what nightmares are made of and I would know because I was the one who was there when they took you from me. You once told me you used to watch scary movies before you would go to sleep in hopes of dreaming about the movie instead of your own hell that was created in your head after your dad died. You shared so much of your pain with me about your upbringing and all I felt I could do was hold you tight and encourage you to get help. You were on that path. It was all too much. If you could only see how it's all too much for me now.

Being blamed for your death and rumors about how our very intentional baby isn't yours was hard enough, but then there was being treated like a leper and robbed of going to your funeral. The worst part about all of it was you not being here to wipe my tears. People are dark, I get it. They all just needed someone to blame, and I'm going to get so much shit for this post, but ask me if I care? I've walked through Hell and seen the devil himself and all I could say was "oh, it's you" and keep walking. I hope those confused individuals are reading this now and feeling like they are ready to make a change for themselves instead of knocking me down to feel better. I know the things you shared with me about your family situation and I did my best to accept them, but now I know what you meant. You were right babe. I made the mistake of encouraging you to mend your relationships with them when you didn't want to and I'm sincerely sorry for that. I now see that you were protecting yourself and I pushed you for the sake of the family we were building. I should have trusted your judgment, given the facts. I thought I was doing the right thing and that was my problem. I pushed you to do better since I was desperate to rush our process with the life we chose. We put ourselves in the hot seat to grow up and get it together before the baby came.

Between recovery and your newly found faith, blending families, and our financial state, I saw you become overwhelmed and did my best to encourage you to get out of the house. All you wanted was to be with me. You became consumed and it hurt me. I thought about sharing our text thread publicly since it was already made known of our ups and downs, our fights, and our love. Everyone could see that we weren't perfect but no relationship is. One thing was for sure and that was that people knew we loved each other deeply.

I drew boundaries and you were hanging on by a thread. I understood your desperation for a happy family because I was just as desperate as you. I loved that you thanked me constantly for showing you what it was like to have a family who loved hard and all I can do now is continue to show our son what loving hard is like by walking in faith. We prayed together, we fought dirty, we abused each other at times, but most importantly, we wanted nothing more than to try to be different than what we were exposed to growing up. We knew we wanted change and longed for the cycle to be broken. I know you told me that you'd rather die than live life without me, and it would make me cringe as much as it would make me smile. Of course, all the romance novels and movies we watched taught us that that was the ultimate act of love. Fuck that. No it is not! Me telling you that I would rather walk away from our relationship to keep our child out of a life of drugs and old behaviors was an act of love. It was love for myself and love for our child. I know the ultimatum was too much but I did what I had to do to protect myself.

You were always so stubborn and self-willed but I knew deep down you wanted help. I knew you were afraid to ask and now you don't have to. I know I didn't kill you and your death isn't my fault, but that doesn't mean that all the people who have cursed me don't hurt. Fuck their assumptions. I was the one holding you as we rocked our bodies back and forth crying. I was your hostage and that's the truth. There was no stopping you and you let me walk away with my life.

I know I'm sharing too much but I'd rather speak up than hold it in and let the monsters take me down. You were battling monsters way before I came into your life and I thought I could help save you from them. I thought I could teach you about God so He could help you. I wanted so badly for you to find your inner strength and confidence but you just couldn't see what I saw. You felt like nothing you could do would be good enough and that broke my heart. I know what it's like to have a brain wired that way, but know that I saw something different. We were taking the world by storm and you decided for both of us how the journey would end. Am I angry? Abso-fuckin-lutely. Do I still love you? Without a doubt. I've got our son to raise without you and I'm going to make sure the cycle stops with him. I will mother with all I have learned about the trauma I've endured and how not to project it onto him and teach him how to use his voice. I will show him that he cannot love anyone else unless he first loves himself.

I will forever and always use my voice and take a stand for myself so I don't fall victim. Sure, I've wanted to pull the trigger too and make this all go away, but I didn't. We would lay our heads down at night, and rise in the morning with such gratitude for finding each other, but now you're gone. Whatever your reason for leaving, my tribute is to raise our son and do my very best to protect him from monsters. I will notice any monsters and show him to respect them, know they are there, but teach him how he can release them to God—where they belong.

I have more control over my life than ever before, and given all the torment, I'm not about to pity myself. I wanted nothing more than to be forged in this fire stronger than I was going in. I am going to use our story to help uplift someone who thinks they don't have a fighting chance. At the end of my day, I don't need anyone's approval, and delivering my raw truth was the best thing I could do for myself. I don't need or crave validation for doing the next right thing and I know what is "right" and "wrong" is open for interpretation; however, I live my life by a code of ethics and that's all I need. Having core beliefs is what allowed me to overcome my battles. My days and nights have blended since you left, and now I must turn my grief into love.

Fighting for justice over the awful things that have been done looks like prayer for me. God always knows how things will end, and when I found out that your mother was left by her husband, I knew that her self-righteous attitude would land her alone, drinking at the bottom of the bottle. I knew that Brit would come around and apologize for causing pain, and now that he is Carter and no longer Brit, he and I are closer than ever. God works and I did what He instructed me to do and that was to NOT fight back. We will have the final victory by leading a healthy, happy life with your spirit entangled with ours. I love you Kaden and I'm sorry for your pain and suffering. You are no longer suffering because God has you. Your son will know that his daddy was nothing short of amazing and you will now live on through our beautiful baby boy.

Love, M.K.

I was starting to feel like I could function a bit better with all the yoga and prayer I was doing alongside some pregnancy classes and therapy to ensure that I didn't make any decisions out of hurt. I even started a support group page on FB called "It's not your fault" to showcase my words of encouragement for those who have been to blame for why a loved one committed suicide. I hate the term "committed suicide" because it insinuates that Kaden committed a crime when he didn't. The anger and hurt I felt towards Kaden were very real, but I still had a strong urge to protect his name. Yes, he left me and his son behind, but for reasons bigger than myself, Kaden felt like he couldn't stay. A close friend told me that God had a purpose for Kaden here on Earth and part of that purpose was to gift me a child, something I didn't realize until I began to forgive Kaden for what he had done. No one will ever know the Kaden I experienced when he was alive, living life sober. People knew he was happy with me, and more importantly, I knew he was happy with me even though we fought towards the end of his life. It was Kaden's private battles that held him captive from me and from the light that was robbed of him that night. Whatever the reason he decided to go, I believed in my heart that it wasn't me who took his life, and no one was going to make me feel like did, not even Brit.

Brit had jumped on the bandwagon with everyone and I had to accept that one of my closest friends was now an enemy, ganging up against me. I didn't trust many people in my life after Kaden died, and that included my father. As much as I love the man, his way of showing up for me was not ideal, and it's not like he was quick to ask me how he could be available for me. He was too busy raising his many babies, never mind making time to visit his daughter who was about to have her own baby. I knew I couldn't rely on my dad and mom for the emotional support I needed, so I stood firm in God and kept my hopes up for the way I was fighting for myself. Everything was a waiting game when it came to fighting over financial assets with Kaden's mom through court, but I knew it would be worth the wait if I didn't give up. What better way to wait than to have Rupert come over and give me attention?

I had just celebrated New Year's with Rupert when I got a text from Hunter asking me how I was doing, pushing me to remember the last time he reached out to me was on the car ride home to TX. I had forgotten about Hunter and was quick to respond to let him know I was doing better while thanking him for reaching out. I knew how much Kaden meant to him. I didn't respond to his last message for fear that he was blaming me like all the rest. There were a select few people that were a part of Kaden's life that knew it wasn't my fault like Kaden's great aunt, cousins, and a few of his ex-girlfriends. I knew they all cared about what was happening to me when they reached out to me with their white flags up doing their best to let me know that they meant no harm. I had already lost those closest to me, the last thing I wanted was more ridicule for being a beautiful woman with a reputation who was in love.

Hunter and I had a brief exchange of messages as I went about my day, thinking about all the other men I was texting at the time just as a distraction. I had only been sleeping with Rupert, who I couldn't help but enjoy my time with, and Hunter was the last person I thought I'd turn into a love interest. Rupert was so sweet and thoughtful when he would come over and get me excited for the arrival of my baby boy. He had already gone down this road before so there were a lot of tips and fun facts he offered me as we engaged in celebratory practices a normal couple would do, like casting my belly with paint for a canvas and going over birthing stories. Rupert held a piece of my heart when he showed how much he cared for me and my son. I began to play with the idea of having him in my life post-pregnancy.

One night, I was laying in bed going through my phone to make sure all the photos of Kaden and I were deleted, since it was my way of lessening the torment, when I came across the photos of Kaden holding the rifle that were so predictably saved to my iCloud. I felt sick the moment I saw the darkness come through the photo, and I began to shake with fear as if I were back in our bedroom that night. I started to cry as I scrolled through my contacts, looking for Rupert's name to call him like every other time I'd called him when I was triggered. It wasn't out of the norm for Rupert to talk me through my panic attacks so I felt secure in knowing he was going to answer. The phone rang and rang and I felt like the air was being sucked from my bedroom with each breath. I jumped out of bed and put my snow boots on so I could head out the door and head over to Rupert's for comfort. I had finally gotten my car back in my possession after all the bopping around from city to city and state to state. It was risky to drive with such a big belly but it had to be done. I had to get to Rupert's as fast as I could.

As I pulled into the long dirt driveway I saw one of Rupert's girlfriend's cars parked next to his in the distance, and I knew I was about to overstay my welcome. I slammed on my brakes and stopped halfway to his house before reversing and heading home. My stomach sank to my ass hole and I felt embarrassed for thinking I was the only one he wanted to be with when I knew he had his own romantic affairs outside of ours. We had been progressive enough with each other by being open about sleeping with other people, but still, I felt entitled to have him when I needed him, and that just wasn't the case.

I sobbed the whole way home and crawled back into bed while chanting out loud, "God help me!" I wanted the vision of Rupert inside another woman out of my head no different than the picture of Kaden's lifeless body out of my head. The haunting of those men had me antsy and ready to end my life as I thought about Zieya hanging herself in a closet. I grabbed one of my scarves and wrapped it tightly around my neck. I went to test the bar in my closet to make sure it could hold my pregnant body when I heard my phone go off. It was Hunter. I stepped out of my closet and went to look at the text Hunter sent me. It was a simple "How are you doing?"

I swiftly responded "Not well," and he offered to call me. When I answered the phone I was doing my best to fool him like I hadn't been crying when he shared with me that I could cry if I needed to. Hunter held space for me to tell him what had been going on with me in that moment of wanting to take my life and not feeling brave enough to do it, or cowardly enough to do it. No matter which way you want to spin it, I couldn't come down from the thought of wanting to die. Hunter then began to walk me through a step-by-step calming technique that had me visualizing myself from outer space, then zooming in on the Earth, then the United States, then on the state I was in, then in my bedroom as I finally found a steady breathing rhythm. I was in awe of how he handled my upset and impressed by his technique that I had never heard of before. I thanked him for sharing some positive reinforcement and let him continue to share positive memories of him and Kaden and their lives growing up. Hunter had offered to share the stories with my son when he was old enough about who his dad was since he and I shared a deep love for Kaden. I never would have thought that Hunter could add to my healing by offering me such compassion as Kaden's best friend.

I was approaching my due date and keeping myself busy by scheduling appointments with my Dula, meeting with my MFM (maternal-fetal medicine) team, and talking to Hunter. It was made known that the females in my family had all struggled with giving birth naturally, and I was starting to get nervous about my birthing plan. Ever since the night I went over to Rupert's I had been keeping my distance from him so he could...do him. I was preoccupied with Hunter anyway and it seemed to me that Hunter was a better version of Rupert. They shared the same profession and rode crotch rockets, they even shared the same musical skill set of playing the drums. I had been so in love with Rupert's musical talents at one point that I sold my brother's stolen motorcycle to buy Rupert a drum set. The most interesting fact these two gentlemen shared was that they were both addicts. Hunter was still sober and working on himself, so it made for some relief when he told me he had over a year of clean time. I learned my lesson by getting involved with anyone who hadn't been at least a year clean.

Hunter and I had finally made plans to hang out together but I was quick to cancel when I found out that I was getting some money after Kaden's property was assessed. After the paternity test, the courts ruled in favor of me and my son, but it was a grim reminder of the hell I was going through with Kaden being gone. I didn't want Hunter to see me down (even though he had heard me cry plenty of times). I would usually seize an opportunity for a guy to see me cry but this time was different. Hunter was not going to take "No" for an answer and insisted on driving 45 minutes away, in a snowstorm, just to cheer me up. When he stomped the snow off his shoes before walking in, I already had butterflies in my stomach and he and I were alone together. For once, I wasn't envisioning his body on top of mine or looking at him like I was going to eat him alive; I simply admired his face and inspected his body language as he helped me around the house.

"Hey M.K."

"Hey what?"

"I've got a surprise for you. I thought it might cheer you up."

"What is it?"

"Grab your coat and let's go for a ride."

I bundled up and excitedly sat in the front seat of his car while he politely asked me to navigate him somewhere deserted. My curiosity switched to nervousness when I asked him, "Why a deserted place?" He then reached into the back seat to grab a tube or a launcher. I smiled at him and asked, "Are we really going to light fireworks right now?"

He responded "Only the good fireworks," as we drove off. We got to a chunk of land flat enough for Hunter to set the launcher down and properly load the mortar shell. I stepped out of his car and rushed to him as he ran to find a spot to light the firework. I yelled out with a jovial tone, telling him to hurry in fear that we would get caught, when I saw the tiniest of sparks fade into the tube. Within seconds, the loudest boom erupted in the night sky. Hunter made it back to the car in time to stare at all the embers floating from the giant BANG! He wasn't joking when he said he got the good kind of fireworks because that sucker was loud, bright, and simply phenomenal. We climbed back in the car after he lit off a second one, pulled out of the dirt parking lot, and headed back to my place. I had never had anyone light off fireworks just to cheer me up, and that's exactly what it did. I was smiling from ear to ear as we got home to finish the night off by playing games and listening to music.

Hunter was super attentive to me by reading Dr. Suess to my belly and he helped me with my low blood sugar by rushing downstairs to grab me some strawberries to remedy my symptoms. It was during a moment of stuffing strawberries in my face that I offered Hunter to stay the night in case he didn't want to make the long trip home. He replied "Yes." I told him I didn't mind him sleeping in my bed with me if he didn't want the couch as I quickly interjected myself with the thought of "We aren't going to have sex," telling Hunter that I was not going to sleep with him no matter how cute I thought he was. We shared some giggles and he respectfully said he didn't mind sleeping on the couch one bit. I thought to myself how familiar his mannerisms were and I had a flash of Kaden's face come through. Hunter reminded me so much of Kaden, and it was no wonder I'd be attracted to him now; they mirrored each other in the strangest of ways.

It was bedtime, and before Hunter said goodnight, I asked him to stay in the bed with me and watch a movie until I fell asleep. It had been my way of soothing, so Hunter got comfy and laid on the right side of the bed, closest to the door. I had fallen asleep when I woke up to darkness and Hunter passed out next to me. I had to pee so I waddled to the bathroom. On my way back to the room I heard Hunter move around, so I thought he was awake too. I climbed back into bed and whispered to him, "Can you hold me?"

Hunter replied "Yes," and scooted his body over to mine. He was the big spoon and I was the little spoon with an even littler spoon as he cupped my pregnant belly. We both fell back to sleep only to wake up from the sweetest moment of affection. Hunter had to work that day so he was up early. Before we said our goodbyes, I made it known how grateful I was for him but how I was in no position to date anyone. Hunter nodded with understanding and hugged me goodbye.

For the next several days, I contemplated my life with Hunter in it but was still so scrambled over my feelings towards Rupert. I was confused as to which man I was going to let be in my life and how I was going to place them in my life once my son was born. Were they going to just be friends with benefits? Or were they going to be the guys on the other end of my texts because I wouldn't want either of them to meet my son? As badly as I wanted a man with me in the delivery room, I couldn't weave any more possibilities over Hunter or Rupert so I let a new state of fear creep in with thoughts of having the baby surgically removed rather than giving birth naturally. What if that's how I died? Would I give birth to my boy so he could live on and I, in turn, could finally meet my maker? I started to play the what-if game as I packed my bag for the hospital and waited for my mom to arrive. Since the world was still at the height of the pandemic, my mom was the only other person allowed to accompany me in the delivery room. Not like I had much of a selection of people to choose from. So, my mom and I checked ourselves into the hospital for my scheduled induced delivery.

Everything in my bones was telling me that I was going to be the break in the chain with how I birthed my child. I was already trend-setting by bringing some dark subjects to my family's attention after Kaden died that they wouldn't have otherwise talked about. I was optimistic and ready for action. Hunter had been texting me and I was sending him cute hospital pics before I started going into labor and things started to take a turn. I prayed before I was doped up by nurses and continued to pray as the doctor had me sign a waiver about using emergency procedures to deliver my baby as the room went silent. The deafness came back to me like every other time I was in the midst of a traumatic event. There was blood everywhere; eight nurses surrounded the doctor as he sat at the foot of my body with my legs spread. My mom was holding my hand, and all I could see was the worry in her eyes and under her masked face as she told me to hang on.

I felt like I was carrying the weight of the world on my organs, and all of a sudden it was gone. A sense of relief had come over me but I hadn't heard any crying. I looked over to the right of me and saw a baby being rushed to a table where a breathing mask was put over his blue face by a nurse. Another nurse surrounded him, blocking my sight of the baby boy I had just delivered. My hearing came back and that's when a nurse asked me if I was ready because she was going to push on my abdomen. Before I could answer, two hands pushed down on me as if she were performing CPR on a 250-pound man. I let out a scream and looked down to see more nurses covered in blood doing their best to maintain the mess.

"She's hemorrhaging, giver her some more Pitocin." I looked over at the many cords I was hooked up to. I hadn't wanted any drugs like Fetanayl in the epidural, so the fear of having anything pumped through my veins left me paralyzed.

I looked at my mom and faintly asked her what was happening when she said "Look." As I turned my head, a nurse was bringing over my revived baby boy. I wasn't able to hold him but they did put him on my chest briefly before taking him back to the NICU (Neonatal Intensive Care Unit) where he was hooked up to monitor after monitor with tubes and cords entering and exiting his 7 pounds 8-ounce body. After the *Carrie* scene was cleaned up, my doctor pushed more paperwork in my face to sign for a blood transfusion to help ensure the safety of my life. I knew that I had just been pushing for three hours and had never felt such pain in my life, so I wasn't in my right mind when I first refused his recommendation. This was my chance to die and be reunited with Kaden, my one true love, my one and only, the only man who loved me so much that he felt he needed to protect me from himself.

What is the perfect love anyway? I knew what it wasn't, and it wasn't judging a book by its cover or taking offense to anything and everything. It wasn't purposely being offensive or pinning others to be the bad guy in hopes you come out the hero. Love wasn't me forcing my way through others' lives in order to get my way. Now that I am a mom, a Christ believer, and a survivor, I think I know what love is. The perfect love for me came to my arms on the fifth day in the hospital and two pints of blood later. After doctors and nurses saved my and my baby's life, I knew that we could keep going and find a way to be happy, together, just him and I. It wasn't a matter of finding the perfect love but of realizing that I had it within me all along. I just needed a lifetime of pain to bring me to my knees before God so He could help reveal how I could love myself and be loved by Him.

To me, that's the whole premise of life: you can't unsee anything you see, and you can't unknow something you know. It's what we do with all these imprints on our hearts and minds that will lead us to the answer to our own happiness. As badly as I wish I could push a delete button, I would have robbed myself of the free will to make a decision about what I've seen and what I've learned. God gave me the free will to make a choice, and each time I walked away with my life, I thanked Him for my self-awareness to make that choice. I am no longer the victim, but a warrior who is ready to fight. Acceptance and boundaries were only taught to me by a loving God. After I went crazy with people pleasing, I went nuts with boundary setting. It was when I held my son for the first time that I let the balance of the two teach me how to be happy in the moment. Being present with my son and accepting my reality was how I was able to commit to being a mother, no different than the commitment it took to be five years sober, no different than waking up every day and identifying as Christian, and certainly no different than making a choice to forgive myself and others for the harm that had been caused. Now there was only one more thing to face—my skincrave.

I went home and stared at my beautiful baby boy and thought about all the mothers of my lovers and thanked them silently for being an example of the kind of mother I didn't want to be. Am I delulu[1] for thinking that I am going to be better than any parenting style I have ever known? We'll see. It's up to me to break the silence around things that should be spoken about. I will be the best mother to my child and I will do it with mindfulness. I want my child to see that his mom isn't ashamed of being who she is, even if it means that I am a sex/love addict, thinking about Hunter being a part of our lives. Should I let him meet my son? My baby boy is the most precious thing to me, and all because I wanted to fulfill a dream of starting a family, this boy is entering a world with no father. Am I wrong for wanting him to have two parents? Can I really raise him by myself? A mix of desperation and protection swirled my thoughts when I heard a knock. I coddled my babe tightly in my arms as I walked towards my front door.

I saw Hunter standing with his blue eyes, dark hair, and his hands in his pockets asking me, "Can I come in?" My heart was beating a melody only my child could understand as I thought to myself, "If I let him in, there is no going back," and I stepped out of the doorway and shut the door.

---

[1] Slang term meaning "delusional"

LEARN ABOUT HEALTHY SEX!

Get plugged in and deepen your level of understanding around SEX
& LOVE addiction. Follow me on:
www.instagram.com/she_is_warriorhybrid
www.linkedin.com/in/mkskincrave00
mkskincrave@gmail.com
And get a free consultation with me for spiritual coaching!

Is your sex life causing more unhealthy habits
rather than promoting security?

Are you left empty after physically and
emotionally pouring into others?

Take a moment to ask yourself these hard questions and you might
discover how you want to handle things differently. Follow me as I
help you put the beauty back in sex and teach you how you can
protect yourself to be mentally, psychically, and spiritually well while
you engage with others!

Learn about sex addiction through SLAA
(Sex and Love Addicts Anonymous)
by finding a meeting near you or

Take my questionnaire at www.tiktok.com/@mkrave00 and
never stop saying SEX!

About the Author

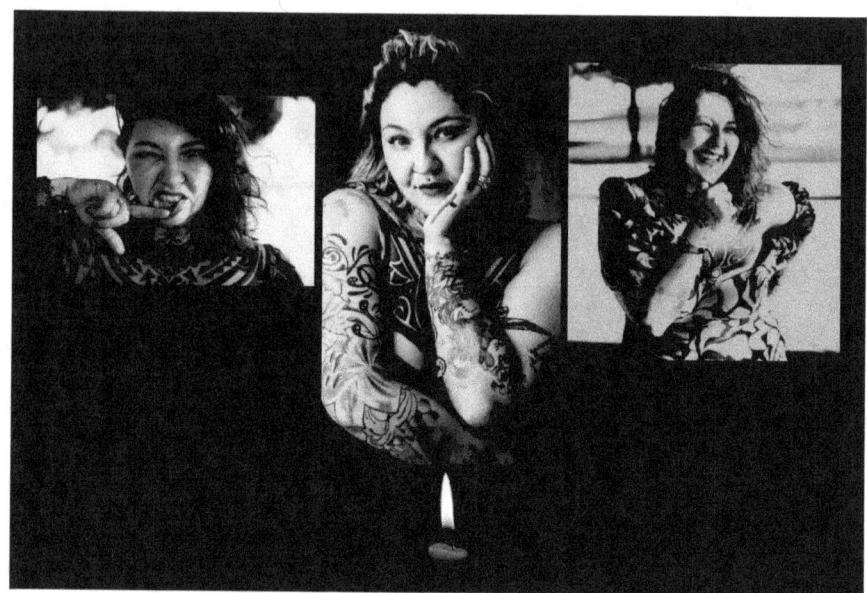

Photo Credit: Daniel Quat of Daniel Quat Photography and Briana Brown of Amarillo Fellowship

M.K. Rave is my pen name. My real name is Megan Kathleen Balizer and I identify as a badass female whose preferred pronouns are her/she. I'm also an addict and a follower of Christ. I get that it is an anomaly for most because of the way I look or how I speak, but I'm here to be the perfect example that I am loved no matter what. I definitely don't mind getting my hands dirty to stand my ground for my beliefs or to advocate for others when they call on me. I'm loud and eccentric and, for me, it's not an impressive resume of accolades that matters, instead hyping up the misfits who are college dropouts like me and chasing their dreams that I care about.

I'm 32 years old and I have used my passions for dance, modeling, theatre, and writing to lead my path outside of my hometown of Santa

Fe, New Mexico. I found myself to be cultured and educated by a school money couldn't buy. The world around me has been my greatest teacher and it would be during my travels that I discovered my desire to be of service. I am now a mother of two beautiful children and they have been my greatest teachers to date. After many years of struggling with active addiction, I would find refuge in a church that would be my pipeline to help others and find my own spiritual walk into fully accepting that I wasn't God. By letting my nomadic lifestyle lead the way, I came across many relationships I would forge love out of and learn about codependency with romance.

My entire love career would speak volumes of how much heartache and beauty are credited for shaping my life. Being a sex and love addict took me overseas, next door, and to my own home until I finally decided enough was enough. Healing the wounds that both myself and others created was the endgame for me, and now that I have children of my own, I want them to have the knowledge I didn't and address the qualms around love and sex. It is a balancing act that I am constantly performing to keep my mental and spiritual health in alignment with the hard truths about my past. My entire journey will play the biggest role in how I raise good humans who aren't afraid to be themselves. I want their self-confidence to exceed in ways that I didn't know how to.